Simplify Your
HEALTH

A DOCTOR'S PRACTICAL GUIDE TO A HEALTHIER LIFE

Martha,

May you have great health!

August, 2022

LUCAS RAMIREZ, MD

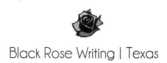

Black Rose Writing | Texas

The author grants the final approval for this literary material.

First printing

This is a work of fiction. Names, characters, businesses, places, events, and incidents are either the products of the author's imagination or used in a fictitious manner. Any resemblance to actual persons, living or dead, or actual events is purely coincidental.

ISBN: 978-1-68513-005-3
PUBLISHED BY BLACK ROSE WRITING
www.blackrosewriting.com

Printed in the United States of America
Suggested Retail Price (SRP) $18.95

Simplify Your Health is printed in Book Antiqua

*As a planet-friendly publisher, Black Rose Writing does its best to eliminate unnecessary waste to reduce paper usage and energy costs, while never compromising the reading experience. As a result, the final word count vs. page count may not meet common expectations.

FOR MY MOM AND DAD,

*I am forever grateful for your
never-ending love and support.
I hope to make you proud.*

Simplify Your
HEALTH

PREFACE

If you ask my mom, she'll tell you she always knew I would end up in medicine. I didn't, though. It had never even crossed my mind. In fact, I started college as an architecture major, but soon found out that my interests and strengths didn't align with that career path. I switched majors to Nutrition Science to complement my passion in athletics. As it turned out, independent of athletics, I found nutrition and biology fascinating, and more so, human anatomy and physiology astounding.

This fascination with the complexity of the human body led me to the medical field. In medical school, we dove deeper into the study of each organ system, of which the nervous system was what most caught my eye. I would visualize the complex circuitry required for mundane tasks. I could see the innumerable chemical interactions required for simple actions such as picking up a pen. Things I never gave thought to now left me in awe. The study of neuroscience drove me to pursue neurology as a career.

My neurology residency was not easy, however. Like many residencies, it involved long hours, busy days, and sleepless nights. I was particularly troubled by my early experiences. I saw many patients with complex neurological conditions who were sick and didn't get better. Patients with neurodegenerative conditions worsened over time, regardless of the medications we gave. I saw patients who were relatively young with

1

devastating neurologic injuries that would forever take away their independence.

The feeling of not being able to help, along with a lack of sleep and 28-hour shifts left me drained, physically and emotionally, eventually leading me to second guess my career choice to the point that I wanted out. I considered leaving medicine altogether, but felt I couldn't do that to my family, who made so many sacrifices to help me reach that point. So I found an alternative (I thought) within medicine, a new residency in Preventive Medicine. I reached out to advisors from my medical school for guidance, searched for programs, and contacted institutions to prepare for a switch.

During this time, I began to see positive changes in the outcomes of patients. I saw patients with major, potentially life-ending strokes get emergent blood clots removed and then do well. Patients with ruptured aneurysms on ventilators, appearing to be at death's door, did remarkably well. I saw one particular patient with a brain bleed, who I didn't expect to regain the ability to talk or walk again, yell at me from a distance in a rehabilitation facility when he saw me. With his wife by his side, and with the help of a cane, he got up from his wheelchair, walked towards me, and thanked me for caring for him in the hospital. These events changed my view of neurology and helped me develop a passion for a subfield within neurology called vascular neurology, which deals with conditions such as strokes, brain bleeds and aneurysms.

My mentor was a vascular neurologist and an important figure in my career development. He frequently gave lectures, and one particular quote has always stuck with me: "80% of strokes can be prevented." This figure came from a 1995 paper published in the *Archives of Neurology* (now the *Journal of the American Medical Association: Neurology*). Though the paper is now dated, that figure is still relevant. The patients I was seeing with strokes were relatively young, in their fifties and sixties, and had many preventable and modifiable risk factors that had directly led to their strokes. I would think to myself, how many of those strokes would have been avoided had they taken care of their health? It was frustrating, to say the least.

My mentor soon gave me the opportunity to speak at community forums, teaching about strokes and the risk factors we can control to prevent them. These experiences motivated me to make stroke prevention—and not just treatment—an important aspect of my future career. I didn't know how I would do it, though I told myself, in some capacity or another, I would.

Which brings me to this point in my life. Today, my career involves the acute treatment of strokes, bleeds, and other neurologic emergencies. However, it doesn't provide me an avenue to *prevent* the very conditions that I treat. Books, however, can bring stories, entertainment, and information to the masses. So, I ventured down this path with the goal of preventing strokes, but soon realized that the risk factors that lead to a stroke also lead to so many other health conditions.

By targeting a few simple lifestyle choices, one can make a world of difference in overall health by decreasing the risks of stroke, heart attacks, cancers and more. One truly has the power to adjust their longevity and quality of life. In this book, I present data from a broad range of source material, different study types, and varying countries of origin, as well as diverse ages and racial demographics of study populations. I also draw data from government agencies, professional organizations, and universities.

Because the data comes from a variety of outlets, it is not all Level 1, Grade A evidence that would meet the scrutiny and standards required to be published in the *New England Journal of Medicine*, for example, but I don't mean it to be. Why? Because this book is not a research article. Instead, it is a compilation of data and information organized and presented to teach, motivate, and inspire action.

Each specific percentage and data point may not apply to you, based on your age and race. But the fact is that humans are very similar to each other. Over 99.9% of your DNA is identical to mine.[1] General findings, then, can be applied to everyone, because habits that are healthy for an individual are going to be healthy (with very rare exceptions) for all humans. And so, I offer substantial data behind my simple recommendations.

I hope you find reading these findings informative, motivating, and entertaining. Most of all, I hope it inspires you to make minor changes that could make a big difference. Because, in all honesty, pursuing health is simple.

Enjoy *Simplify Your Health.*

- Lucas Ramirez, MD
November 2021

1. INTRODUCTION:
OUR BURDEN OF DISEASE

"It is health that is real wealth and
not pieces of gold and silver."
- Mahatma Gandhi

A Reality

On a late Los Angeles night in 2018, my pager went off. I was
then a Stroke Fellow at the University of California, Los Angeles
(UCLA), so a beeping pager could only mean one thing: a stroke
code. Luckily, I was still awake, which made my response time
just a bit faster, and in stroke care, 'time is brain.' In fact, the
typical stroke patient loses nearly 2 million neurons each
minute.[2] I lived close to the hospital, and given the time, there
was no traffic. I arrived quickly with the rest of the stroke
response team to rapidly assess the patient.

She was 70 years old or so, an African American woman who
was out with her girlfriends, singing karaoke, when she
suddenly felt dizzy, had a change in her vision, and collapsed.
Her friends had frantically called 911. The medics found her
unresponsive, with weakness on one side of the body. They
activated the stroke pre-notification system and rushed her to
our facility, where we were ready for her.

The emergency physicians immediately ensured her ABCs were stable (airway, breathing, and circulation). Then we, the neurology team, quickly assessed. We could not do our typical stroke exam because the patient was in a nearly comatose state; her eyes were misaligned, and as we could tell by simply pinching her limbs, she clearly moved one side of the body less than the other. A sudden comatose-like state and asymmetric weakness usually means one of two things: a brain bleed or a dangerous stroke in a critical area of the brain called the brain stem.

We had notified the CT scanner ahead of time, so the unit was open, and we rushed the patient over. A quick scan revealed that there was no bleeding, and the second scan looking at her arteries showed exactly what we expected: an occluded basilar artery. The basilar artery is a major artery supplying blood to the brainstem. This area of the brain is vitally important for regulating breathing, consciousness, and much more; therefore, her condition was life-threatening.

We activated the intervention team and rushed the patient to the angiography suite, where a catheter was placed in her groin, inserted into her femoral artery, and advanced into the basilar artery in her head. Here, a special stent was pushed into the clot, and it opened. Its design allowed it to embed into and grab hold of the clot. It was then pulled out, and thankfully, the clot with it. Within minutes, we restored blood flow to the basilar artery and brain stem. This procedure, called a thrombectomy, has become the standard of care in certain acute stroke syndromes only within the last 10 years, and it has revolutionized stroke care and drastically improved outcomes.

A basilar artery occlusion is typically a devastating type of stroke. When first described in the literature more than 50 years ago, it was assumed to be a fatal diagnosis.[3] With rapid, successful treatment, that is not the case today. After several days under our care, our patient was able to walk out of the hospital without help, and went home with only a slightly drooped smile. It was an amazing case that has stuck in my memory.

Health Defined

The patient from the story above was "healthy" by typical societal norms. She lived independently, didn't require help, and had no major health conditions that impaired her daily life. If health is the combination of a longevity and functionality, then on the surface, she definitely appeared to be healthy. So why would a healthy person suddenly have a potentially catastrophic stroke?

The fact is, we are human, and the inevitable truth that comes with life is aging and eventual death; yet we can delay that ultimate certainty and make those later years better. *We can approach the goal of longevity and functionality like any goal – or inversely, any problem – by looking at the root causes to have a directed target for intervention.* My patient had several risk factors that were not being addressed properly because she was unaware of them. These risk factors were the reasons (or root causes) that her life nearly irreversibly changed. To better understand and address the roots of such problems, let's look at the principal causes of death and disability while also focusing on the major risk factors leading to those conditions. This foundation will lead us to the short list of things we can do to improve our health.

Death and Disability by the Numbers

Despite all our medical advancements, stroke is still a leading cause of disability and death in the United States and worldwide. In the US, the leading causes of death, in order, are: heart disease, cancer, unintentional injuries, chronic obstructive pulmonary disease (COPD), and stroke (Figure 1).[4] These five conditions alone accounted for 61% of all deaths in 2019.[5]

Worldwide, the causes of death, though not identical, are similar. Heart disease is first, followed by strokes, COPD, lower respiratory infections, and lung/airway cancer (Figure 2).[6] Based on these statistics, the US and the world share three (nearly four) of the leading causes of death.

With a more detailed look, one can see that the leading causes change based on the economic profile of a nation. Clear socioeconomic differences worldwide result in unique exposures, nutritional intake, activity levels, and healthcare infrastructure for a population. In low-income countries, for example, contagious diseases are more common, while for high-income countries, the leading causes of death nearly mirror those in the US. Regardless of the wealth of a nation and its people, humans are humans, and certain conditions tend to afflict all groups. Of these, heart disease and stroke are the most generalizable and leading killers worldwide, and as the economic strata begins to rise and exposures change, COPD and cancers gain traction.

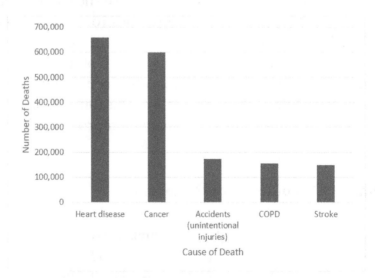

Figure 1: Top 5 leading causes of Death in the US, 2019

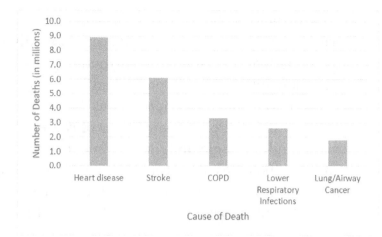

Figure 2: Top 5 leading causes of Adult Death in the World, 2019

Compiling an accurate and unified list of the leading causes of disability is a bit more complicated, in part, because of the ways we define and measure disability. In practical terms, we can consider disability as a condition that impairs a person's ability to engage in tasks and activities. This impairment can be physical (such as inability to move a side of the body) or cognitive (such as inability to express speech). By using the most widespread statistical approach, the leading causes of disability in the US in 2017 were heart disease, lung cancer, COPD, diabetes, and low back pain.[7]

We can compare this data to other methods of measurement to see how applicable this is to everyday life. The Unam Group is a leading provider in disability benefits, covering over 36 million customers[8] with an annual revenue of more than 11 billion dollars.[9] In a review of disability claims, they found that in 2017, the leading causes of long-term disability were cancer, back disorders (back pain), injury, heart disease, and joint disorders.[10] The two lists are similar and suggest that we can reliably use the listed conditions for our ongoing discussion about quality of health and how to achieve it.

Cancer is a pathology that differs from heart disease and stroke. Cancer is simply the abnormal and accelerated division of cells in the body that may spread to surrounding tissues. A detailed discussion into the pathophysiology and the many types of cancer is outside the scope of this book. Yet it is important to know that there are many types of cancers, many causes of cancer, and no single unifying treatment of cancer. In fact, there are over 100 types of cancers affecting all organs and tissue types.[11] In the US, lung cancer accounts for the most cancer deaths, followed by colon/rectum, pancreas, breast and prostate (Figure 3).[12]

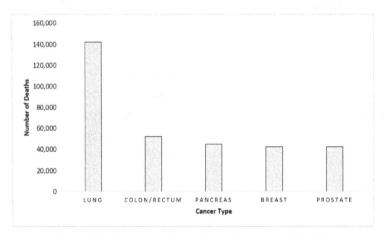

Figure 3: Leading Causes of Cancer-Related Deaths in the US in 2018

The data presented points to vascular diseases (including heart disease and stroke) and cancers as leading causes of death and disability in the US and worldwide. Now that we have identified our problems, we must look at the root causes. Next, I give an easy example of a root cause analysis.

Finding the Roots

The California earthquake of 1906 destroyed much of San Francisco. The immediate destruction itself occurred because of collapsed buildings and fires, though the common reason for the collapses and fires in the first place was the major earthquake, which was the actual root cause of all the destruction. So, what are the actual root causes of the diseases harming us?

We can look at this in two parts: causes we cannot change and causes we can change. I cannot change my age or genetics. Somebody in their seventies (like my patient with the basilar artery clot) is going to have a higher chance of a heart attack compared to someone in their twenties. That is a non-negotiable fact. What I *can* change are my habits and behaviors. These are modifiable. *This modification is the key.* **The root causes we are interested in are the modifiable risk factors that can lead to the diseases causing the most death and disability, because *we can* change these risks.** So, let's look at the root causes of the major diseases afflicting us.

More than 50% of cardiovascular disease in a US population could be explained by only five modifiable risk factors.[13] These are:

- high blood pressure,
- diabetes,
- smoking,
- high cholesterol, and
- obesity.

The most impactful of these is high blood pressure, which accounted for 25% of all cardiovascular events.[13] This was exactly what my patient had without knowing it, and it was the major risk leading to her stroke. Globally, a staggering 90% of strokes result from poorly controlled modifiable risk factors.[14] The aforementioned risk factors attributing to cardiovascular disease also influence cancer. Smoking is the number one risk factor for lung cancer, and is linked to 80 to 90% of all lung cancer deaths.[15] It additionally accounts for eight out of ten COPD deaths.[16] Obesity is associated with a higher risk of breast cancer. Being overweight or obese accounts for 16% of postmenopausal breast cancers.[17]

The True Causes of Our Disease

Although these risk factors are not the ultimate causes of death in and of themselves, they are linked, and, in large part, the direct causative factor leading to the development of the diseases which cause death and disability. Thus, they may be seen as the "true" causes. This concept has garnered a growing amount of data. In 2005, smoking and high blood pressure were the leaders, accounting for one in every five to six deaths in US adults, followed by being overweight or obese and physically inactive, with each responsible for nearly one in ten deaths. A combination of poor dietary habits (poor diet) rounded out the list of "true" causes of death (Figure 4).[18] In a later analysis, the leading causes of "actual" death in the US in 2010 were poor diet and physical inactivity, smoking, and alcohol consumption.[19]

This isn't just an American phenomenon. The root causes of death on a global scale follow a similar pattern. An analysis found that the risk factors driving the most death worldwide in 2017 were high blood pressure, smoking, high sugars, air pollution, and obesity.[20] Just like roots which lead to the trunk of a tree, our basic root cause analysis leads us to a short-list of the most impactful reasons that we develop the diseases that cause our death and disability. These include smoking, high blood pressure, poor diet, physical inactivity, obesity, and alcohol consumption.

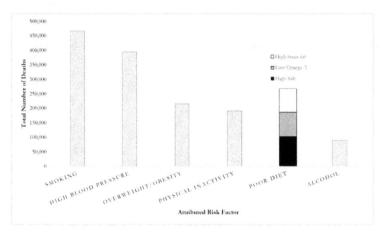

Figure 4: True Causes of Death in the US in 2005

Achieving Health

So, what is health, and how can we achieve it? From my perspective, **health is the combination of years of life, the quality of those years, and the control of risk factors that lead to the development of our major health conditions.** In the US (as of 2010), nearly 20% of the population still smokes, 30% have high blood pressure, over 35% are obese, and nearly 50% do not meet physical activity goals. These are all modifiable conditions that are addressable both at the individual and population levels.[21]

There is no shortage of steps one can take to improve individual health, and the list of things to change in our daily lives can be extensive and even impossible to implement. To make them more manageable, we can compress the enormous list of ways to be healthy to the most impactful interventions that are realistically achievable and practical to implement. I will detail eight steps to improve health, and, importantly, show why these steps are so impactful. These are:

-Do not smoke
-Drink only in moderation
-Pursue a healthy weight
-Increase physical activity
-Improve your eating habits
-Check your blood pressure
-Get recommended screenings
-Get vaccinated

I will split this information into two sections. The first requires no external help; it's just you and your behaviors. The second involves the external help of someone other than you, namely, your doctor. A brief summary of these actions can be found at the end, but as they say, "knowledge is power," and so the bulk of this book provides knowledge about why the changes work, with the goal of instilling power and motivation to successfully make changes to your daily habits.

To summarize, much of our disease burden is rooted in key risk factors. This emphasis on key risk factors will be the backbone of this book and of the chapters. I will expand upon each risk factor. Importantly, interventions will be provided and summarized in short, immediately applicable ways.

Now that we have our targets for intervention, we can proceed to the first step toward better health.

SECTION 1:
CHOICES ONLY YOU CAN MAKE

"Our bodies are our gardens,
to which our wills are our gardeners."
- William Shakespeare

2. DO NOT SMOKE

"I haven't had a cigarette in 6 years ...
that's because I'm scared of my wife."
- Former US President Barack Obama

Tobacco through History

In November 1492, Christopher Columbus documented is his diary: "...men and women with firebrand of weeds in their hands to take in the fragrant smoke to which they are accustomed." It was the first documented encounter between Europeans and tobacco in the Americas. Tobacco smoking was subsequently introduced upon the expedition's return to Spain, and eventually became fashionable and spread throughout Europe.[22]

In the US, tobacco has been popular since at least the Colonial Era. In the late 1880s, about 56% of the tobacco consumed was as chewing tobacco, while only 1% was from cigarette smoking.[23] Once the production of cigarettes became mechanized, cigarette use soared. In 1900, the average US adult smoked 54 cigarettes annually, this increased to 4,345 cigarettes (over half a pack per day) by 1963.[23] Tobacco use peaked in the 1960s, when over 40% of US adults smoked. The glamor of smoking in movies, television and advertising campaigns drove the exponential rise.[23] Consumption markedly decreased since the 1960s following the publication of the harmful effects of cigarette smoking by the first Surgeon General's report, and the subsequent tobacco control polices and increases in antismoking societal norms.[23]

Smoking is Evolving

Although the overall trends are promising, there is still a substantial burden of smoking today. Fourteen percent of US adults, over 34 million people, are currently cigarette smokers.[24] Among teens, 6% of high school students smoke cigarettes.[25] There are about 16.8 million high school students in the US,[26] equating to over 1 million high school students who smoke. What's worse, the use of any tobacco product has increased over the past decade, largely driven by electronic cigarette use.[27] In 2019, 28% of high school students (4.7 million) were using e-cigarettes. That is a massive increase of over 1,700% compared to 2011.[27] Smoking is not confined to traditional and electronic cigarettes; 8% report smoking cigars, 3% hookahs, and 1% pipes.[25] Although a non-tobacco product, 22% of high school seniors report smoking marijuana;[28] that's more than cigarettes, cigars, hookahs, pipes and binge drinking combined; and the rate of daily use is increasing.[28]

The rate of marijuana use has also risen in adults.[29] In fact, 14% of US adults, over 34 million people, report regular marijuana use.[30] That is the same as those reporting current cigarette use. The burden of smoking any product, not just cigarettes, remains significant, and the decreasing trends of use we've seen in decades past are being stifled by a rise in smoking alternate products. All these have their unique risks, but all have a commonality (aside from electronic cigarettes) in the inhalation of combustion byproducts, which results in a shared risk.

Combustion

Combustion is a chemical process in which fuel combines with oxygen and gives off heat.[31] Fire is the visible effect of combustion.[32] Fuel for combustion can be in the form of a gas, liquid, or solid (such as wood, coal, tobacco or marijuana).[32] Incomplete combustion from burning solids results in fire and smoke along with many byproducts that are health-damaging pollutants.[32,33] Getting technical, these include inorganic gases (like carbon monoxide), hundreds of hydrocarbons and oxygenated inorganics (which can cause cancer), free radicals, and particulate matter (which cause oxidative stress and inflammation).[33] Smoke, and the chemicals in it, come into contact with the mouth, nose, throat and lungs, where it then diffuses into the bloodstream and reaches organs. Thus, inhalation of smoke potentially increases the risk of cancer wherever blood is taken to, and that's everywhere in the body, with the greatest risk occurring in the respiratory tract.

Free radicals and fine particles in smoke can lead to irritation and inflammation in the lungs, resulting in both short-term and long-term lung injury.[34] Damage to the artery wall speeds plaque formation in the arteries of our bodies, a process known as atherosclerosis. Free oxygen radicals damage our artery walls, leading to the deposition of cholesterol and other secondary reactions which cause plaque buildup. If this occurs in the heart, it can lead to heart attacks, and in the brain, it can lead to strokes. Taken together, both are the major components of cardiovascular disease.

We can see the effects of smoke inhalation from the combustion of *any* carbon-containing product. Forest and brush fires lead to increased emergency room visits for asthma, COPD, bronchitis, laryngitis, sinusitis, and other upper respiratory infections.[33] Residential wood burning, like that for home heating, results in systemic inflammation and increases the risk of wheezing, cough, sore throat, serious lung infections, and asthma exacerbations.[33] Exposure to indoor combustion is higher in undeveloped countries compared to the US, and the data regarding the risks of this exposure is readily available. Half of the world's households still cook with solid fuels daily, [33] and studies have showed an increased risk of pneumonia, low birth weight, stillbirth, COPD, lung cancer, blindness from cataracts, and cardiovascular disease.[33,35]

As we can see, there are clear and shared mechanisms by which smoke inhalation can lead to negative health effects. In modern America, the most likely source of smoke inhalation is from cigarettes, and more recently, the rising use of marijuana. Electronic cigarettes do not use combustion, and their health effects are independent of what we discussed regarding smoke and particulates. What follows is a more detailed look at the consequences of these three major sources of smoking.

Traditional Cigarettes: An Overview

As we've seen, smoking tobacco as cigarettes has decreased substantially since the 1960s, though it continues to be of significance in the US. Smoking is a major risk factor for many diseases, and over 480,000 annual deaths are directly attributed to the complications of smoking. That is one in every five deaths in the US.[36] In fact, it is the deadliest modifiable behavior and the leading cause of preventable death in the US.[36] Globally; the burden is massive. Over the course of the twentieth century, estimations suggest that tobacco smoking has killed around 100 million people.[37] In 2017 alone, it resulted in over 7 million deaths.[37] Again; it is the deadliest behavioral risk factor and the second deadliest modifiable risk factor, only behind high blood pressure. Some estimates suggest that one billion deaths during the twenty-first century will be attributed to smoking tobacco.[37]

So why is smoking such a lethal habit? Well, besides the effects related to combustion, nicotine and tobacco (independent of combustion) have biological side effects resulting in negative health consequences.

The Impact of Nicotine and Tobacco

Nicotine exerts its effect through stimulation of specific nicotine receptors in the brain, nervous system, and target organs (such as the inner lining of blood vessels, muscles, skin, kidneys, and lungs).[38] The addictive potential of nicotine is common knowledge, though the additional effects are not as commonly known. The nicotine receptors appear to trigger cellular pathways involved in the promotion of cancer and facilitation of metastasis.[38] Nicotine also appears to promote plaque progression in atherosclerosis (commonly known as hardening of the arteries).[38] It also appears to suppress cellular immunity, including the production of antibodies, which can impair the body's defenses against infectious organisms.[38] There is also evidence that nicotine has adverse effects on reproductive health, including preterm delivery, stillbirth and adverse effects on fetal lung and brain development.[38]

Milder adverse effects of nicotine include nausea and vomiting, progressing to diarrhea, excess salivation, excess lung secretions, and decreased heart rates. High doses of nicotine can also lead to acute toxic effects. Severe intoxication can lead to seizures and decreased breathing.[38] It can even be fatal, though the dose is not clearly defined. A reported dose of 50 to 60 mg is "poorly documented," and "no study was located as a source for an estimate of the dose that is fatal to humans."[38] I emphasize here that it is unclear if the reported lethal dose is accurate, though to put this dose in perspective, it's about the same as the sudden use of about 30 low dose Nicorette gums,[39] 60 cigarettes,[40] or three Juul pods.[41]

In contrast, the negative effects of tobacco are widely known because of public education campaigns, so we will only briefly touch upon that information here. Tobacco smoke is made of thousands of chemicals, including at least 70 known to cause cancer.[42] Some cause heart disease, lung disease, and other health effects. Many of these are completely independent of combustion and are in the tobacco itself, including tobacco-specific nitrosamines, benzo[a]pyrene, and other polycyclic aromatic hydrocarbons.[42] We find these in smoked and smokeless tobacco products. The biological effects of smoke, tobacco, and nicotine make cigarettes toxic to the body, leading to a wide range of health effects.

Negative Health Effects of Cigarette Smoking

The list of health effects caused by tobacco is extensive: heart disease, stroke, COPD, cancer (lung, bladder, blood, colon, rectum, esophagus, kidney, ureter, larynx, liver, oropharynx, pancreas, stomach, trachea, bronchus), reduced fertility, pregnancy-related adverse effects (preterm delivery, stillbirth, miscarriages, low birth weight, ectopic pregnancy, cleft palate, birth defects), sudden infant death syndrome, effects on bone health, tooth loss, gum disease, eye disease (cataracts, age-related macular degeneration), decreased immune function, rheumatoid arthritis, and more.[43] We can focus on a select few to illustrate its impact.

As mentioned before, four of the five leading causes of death in the US are heart disease, cancer, COPD, and stroke. Smoking is powerfully related to them all. From 2005 to 2009, smoking lead to the annual death of nearly 125,000 people from heart disease, over 160,000 from cancer, over 100,000 from COPD, and over 15,000 from stroke.[36] In 2009, these four diseases caused more than 1.4 million deaths in the US,[44] and 28% resulted from the effects of cigarette smoking. This doesn't even include the 41,000 who died from secondhand smoke.[36] The effects are strongest for lung cancer and COPD. Smoking causes about 90% of all lung cancer deaths and 80% of all deaths from COPD.[43] It's estimated that if no one smoked, one of every three cancer deaths in the US would not occur.[43]

Although not as strongly causal as the two earlier findings, 21% of strokes[14] and about 13% of heart disease[13] are attributed to smoking. Compared to a non-smoker, smokers have four times the risk of heart disease, four times the risk of stroke, and twenty-five times the risk of lung cancer.[43] Clearly, smoking is devastating to the body.

I often hear people say, "I only smoke occasionally," as a way of justifying their smoking habit. It leads to the reasonable question: how many does one have to smoke to have these consequences? We can look at the question with indirect and direct data, the former having abundant data as second-hand smoking. Studies show that just *being around* smoke makes people more likely to get cancer and cardiovascular disease. Nonsmokers who breathe in secondhand smoke at home or work increase their risk of developing heart disease by 25 to 30% and stroke by 20 to 30%.[45] Secondhand smoke exposure causes over 7,300 lung cancer deaths each year.[46] The concentration of smoke in offices, restaurants, or apartment complexes inhaled by secondhand smokers is clearly far lower than that of direct smokers, showing that even a nominal amount of tobacco smoke is harmful.

Quantifying exactly how much smoking is required to cause what disease severity is a complex task. Lab studies suggest that "no level of smoking or exposure to secondhand smoke is safe."[47] At the lowest detectable levels of exposure, smoking can induce changes in genetic expression in the linings of airways,[47] which may lead to lung diseases. Observational data shows that people who smoke less than one cigarette per day had a nine times greater risk of premature death from lung cancer and a 64% increased risk of premature death from any cause as compared to people who never smoke.[48] Even occasional smoking was found to be associated with a 60% increased risk of early death in men.[49]

Based on these findings, NO LEVEL OF SMOKING IS SAFE, whether for a heavy daily smoker, a light smoker, or an occasional smoker. The good news is that smoking rates have decreased in the US over that last half century, leading to about a 40% decrease in male cancer death rates, and the prevention of at least 146,000 lung cancer deaths from 1991 to 2003.[50] Unfortunately, recent years have also seen a rise in alternate smoking products, one of which was touted as a means of quitting tobacco, but is instead leading to a new generation of smokers: those who use electronic cigarettes.

Electronic Cigarettes: An Overview

While there had been a slow and steady decline in the rates of cigarette smoking for decades, in recent years, there has been steep incline in the use of e-cigarettes, especially among youth. While cigarette smoking in high schoolers decreased over 50% between 2011 and 2017, e-cigarette use increased 1733% between 2011 and 2019.[27] A product that is supposedly "designed for adult smokers looking to move away from traditional cigarettes"[51] is now being used en masse by young people who had never smoked before. This epidemic of e-cigarette use amongst youth is worrisome for two reasons: the risks of using and the risks of becoming traditional cigarette users. We'll first discuss the former risk.

Health Effects of E-Cigarettes

What are the health risks of e-cigarette use? I would preface this presentation of findings with a caution: this is a relatively new product, and it could take decades to see the long-term risks. For now, however, certain things are clear: e-cigarettes contain nicotine, and we know that nicotine is harmful for the reasons stated earlier in the chapter (including promotion of cancer and metastasis, promotion of plaque progression, suppression of cellular immunity, adverse effects in reproductive health, and acute toxic effects including in its most severe cases, seizures, and even death).

Although only popular for approximately a decade, clinical data is already showing negative effects of e-cigarettes, despite vaporizing technologies eliminating the risks of combustion.[52] E-cigarettes have been found to increase metabolism in the spleen and blood vessels, speeding up the development of atherosclerosis and plaque buildup.[53] This can lead to clinical consequences. Data suggests that compared with non-users, e-cigarette users have higher odds of both strokes and heart attacks.[54] There also is an association with seizures, as more than 100 seizures and other neurological problems linked to vaping products have been reported to the Food and Drug Administration (FDA) during the last decade,[55] possibly related to nicotine.

In addition, even though e-cigarette technology eliminates the need for combustion, the aerosolized vaper is *not* harmless. The fluids contain at least seven groups of potentially toxic compounds,[56] and the resulting vapor can contain harmful substances such as nicotine, flavoring chemicals (linked to serious lung disease), cancer-causing chemicals, and heavy metals (such as lead).[57] Studies show that the aerosol causes injury to the small airways of the lungs.[58] Thus, one can expect lung diseases to occur because of this habit. Use of these products increases the odds of a chronic cough, phlegm, and bronchitis.[58] In its most serious form, the inhaled aerosol can cause an acute chemical lung injury termed e-cigarette or vaping–associated lung injury (EVALI). As of January 2020, 2,711 patients have been hospitalized with EVALI with 60 confirmed deaths.[56] Most cases involved delta-9-tetrahydrocannabinol (THC) or cannabidiol (CBD) containing liquid, formulated with oils such as vitamin E. Seventeen percent though didn't contain THC nor CBD, and only used nicotine vaping products.

We are also seeing data linking vaping products to cancer. A recent study showed that mice exposed to e-cigarette vapor containing nicotine had an increased risk of developing lung cancer and pre-cancerous changes in the bladder.[59] There is not enough data to make conclusions about cancer risks in humans; for now, though, the results of lab and animal studies are worrisome.

Besides the health consequences of e-cigarettes themselves, there's a concerning association with traditional cigarette use. As mentioned, e-cigarettes are marketed as a means of quitting smoking for adults, though the exact opposite is occurring. Data suggests that teens who never would have smoked are now vaping.[60] Even worse, e-cigarette use increases the likelihood of smoking cigarettes in young people. Youth in the US are seven times as likely to try cigarettes and eight times as likely to be current cigarette smokers if they previously tried vaping.[58] It's estimated that e-cigarettes are culpable for almost 200,000 new cigarette smokers.[58]

Unfortunately, cigarettes are addicting, and quitting once you start is difficult. More likely than not, a teen smoker will become a long-term smoker. Three out of four teens who smoke end up smoking into adulthood,[61] and nearly 90% of adult smokers began their habit before the age of 18.[62] If someone is already an adult smoker, can vaping help stop the habit? Of US adult smokers trying to quit, about one third attempt to substitute traditional cigarettes with e-cigarettes.[63] A study comparing e-cigarettes to other nicotine products (like gum or patches) showed that e-cigarettes lead to smoking abstinence within one year in 18% of people, compared to 10% for other products. The problem is that at one year, 80% of those with e-cigarettes were still vaping.[64] Thus, the vast majority were smoking and vaping *simultaneously*. This is similar to findings from the CDC showing most adult e-cigarette users do not stop smoking cigarettes and are instead continuing to use both products.[63] The combination is more dangerous than either alone.

The fact is, e-cigarettes are harmful both short- and long-term. It is suggested they are less harmful than traditional cigarettes,[65] and that may be the case. Although long-term data is lacking, we currently know that the liquid that is aerosolized and then inhaled contains chemicals that are dangerous. We also know that we don't fully understand the extent of its effects. Until our knowledge of e-cigarettes catches up with that of traditional cigarettes, it would be prudent to avoid using e-cigarettes as a means of quitting and to focus instead on other methods to help stop smoking.

The Push to Quit

Quitting the habit of smoking is beneficial to health at any age. After one year of quitting, the added risk of heart disease is half that of a continuing smoker. By two to five years, the increased risk of stroke is back to the level of a non-smoker. At five years, the risk of mouth, throat, esophagus, and bladder cancer decreases by 50%. By 10 years without smoking, the risk of lung cancer is half that of a continuing smoker. Finally, at 15 years, the risk of heart disease is back to the level of a non-smoker.[66] Thus, any time is a good time to quit.

This fact is not lost on the general population. A majority (about 68%) of smokers want to quit.[67] The problem is that it is much easier said than done. In 2018, 55% of smokers reported trying to quit, with only 7.5% successfully quitting over the year.[67] Thus, about five in ten smokers try, and one in ten smokers succeed. So, what can help someone successfully quit the habit? Everyone is unique, and one method does not fit all; however, one can look at the advice and studies of those who have done so successfully.

First, a person needs a true motivation and desire to quit. There are many reasons people decide to quit cigarettes. Health is clearly one reason, which I have tried to cement in the mind of you, the reader. Ideally, one should strive to quit prior to developing health consequences. A smoking ban at home or at work is an important motivator for quitting.[68] A significant other can play an important role. For example, smoking may not be allowed at home because a wife is pregnant, or because there is a child in the house. These can be powerful deterrents. Cost is another important factor.[68] The average pack of cigarettes in California is $8.31.[69] Thus, a pack-per-day smoker would spend $3,033 per year on the habit.

I had a patient with erectile dysfunction because of arterial disease, in large part caused by smoking. He used brand-name Viagra when intimate with his wife, but he complained of the cost. That "little blue pill" was about $450 dollars per six tablets.[70] Even with special promotions by Pfizer offering 50% off, that's $225 for six tablets, or about $38 dollars per tablet. I told him that for every week of not smoking, he would save about $55, which would cover one tablet with some extra change. Imagine: not only can quitting the habit fund the pills to improve one's sex life, it can also improve erectile function directly.[71]

Whatever the motivation may be, once it's there, plan ahead and have help and resources available for when you pull the trigger on quitting. What follows summarizes advice from several resources,[72,73,74] intertwined with my personal input.

Choose a quit day, schedule it, and stop on that day. Quitting smoking abruptly is more likely to lead to long-term success compared to a gradual reduction.[75] That's not to say that it will be easy. The majority fail when quitting cold turkey. Using nicotine replacement increases the chance of success by 50 to 60%.[76] Using a nicotine patch along with another form of nicotine (like gum or a lozenge) further increases the chances of success as much as 36% compared to a single nicotine replacement.[77]

Consider using a nicotine patch plus nicotine gum and consider starting them one day before your quit day. Data also suggest that starting nicotine replacement the day before quitting increases the chance of abstinence by 25%.[77] This will help, although quitting will not be a cakewalk.

Many will need additional help to decrease cravings. The FDA has approved 2 non-nicotine smoking cessation medications: Varenicline (marketed as Chantix) and Buproprion (marketed as Zyban). Both are short-term medications used for 12 weeks to help with the early period after quitting. After a 12-week course of Varenicline, quitting for a full year is over 3 times as likely compared to quitting cold turkey, and potentially 40% more likely than with a nicotine patch alone.[78] Adding a second 12-week course further increases the likelihood of quitting by 34%.[78] Bupropion also makes quitting more likely, though when both are compared to each other, Varenicline has marginal benefit.[78] They can be used with nicotine, and heavy smokers may benefit from the combination. Importantly, no increased side effects were reported with the combination.[78]

Thus, for heavy smokers, or those who have tried to quit and failed while using nicotine, consider using Varenicline

more so than Buproprion along with nicotine patches and gum. This is not to say that there are no side effects from these medications. All medications have potential risks, and these are no different. Varenicline can cause nausea, headaches, insomnia, and abnormal dreams.[78] The most commonly reported side effects from Buproprion are insomnia, nausea, vomiting, and dizziness.[79] The severity of is not too significant in either case, since there is no difference in the rates of stopping the medications due to side effects compared to placebo or nicotine.[78,79] Both have been reportedly associated with mood and behavioral disturbances, and even with suicide shortly after starting the medication,[78,79] though these mood disturbances are also observed in patients attempting to quit cold turkey, thus clouding actual correlation with the medication. In 2016, the FDA removed the black box warning for Varenicline, and removed language suggesting serious psychiatric effects from Buproprion as these risks were "lower than previously suspected."[80] I emphasize: please speak with your doctor about your health conditions to see if these, and/or nicotine, are appropriate therapies for you. If so, these should be started about one week before your quit day.

It is important to have support. Even with all the above medications and other options, quitting will not be easy. Tell family and friends of your plans and lean on them for support. There are free expert quit lines for additional help, such as 1-800-QUIT-NOW, though many national and local support groups can be easily found online. If needed, see a counselor in person.

Plan ahead, get an app or journal to document your experience, lean on loved ones, and use quit lines and or counselors for help if needed. As stated earlier, it's important to have a plan, document when you get cravings, identify and remove triggers (such as alcohol and stress) and to find alternate ways to deal with cravings (such as exercise, chewing gum, and brushing your teeth). Modern technology can help with planning. For example, smokefree.gov has resources for smoke-free texting programs, smoke-free social media connections, and recommended apps to help with planning, identifying, and documenting the process (such as QuitGuide and quitSTART). Again, many resources are available online.

There is no harm in finding a good, licensed therapist or acupuncturist for added help. Alterative therapy exists, such as hypnosis and acupuncture, and though little evidence supports its benefits in smoking cessation (per the American Cancer Society), some feel that these methods helped. If you relapse, it's okay. Keep trying, tweak your approach, and use combinations of all the approaches we've reviewed.

Even better than quitting is never starting at all. As stated earlier, a teen smoker will probably become an adult smoker. The vast majority of adult smokers began smoking in their teens. It's imperative for a parent to start a dialogue about smoking early and continue through childhood and teenage years.

Talk about the health risks and the advertising that tries to prey on teens by glamorizing smoking and making it seem "cool" when it is anything but. Discuss how it's not 'rebellious' to smoke; plainly put, it's unhealthy. Talk about peer pressure, something they will face, and how to respond without appearing scared or nervous. Talk about willpower and self-confidence. Talk about the addictive potential, and how most teen smokers continue smoking through adulthood. Talk about the cost and what they can purchase in its place for the same dollar amount. Obviously, I am in no position to tell you, the reader, how to raise your children, but if you do not want your children to smoke, then this approach may help you.

Set boundaries. Do not permit smoking of any product (including e-cigarettes) and prohibit smoking paraphernalia in your home. Be strict about a smoke-free home including with friends and guests.

Most important, set an example. If you are a smoker, quit, or at least try to quit. Talk about your struggles to quit (if you've had them), your cravings, and how that addiction is something to avoid.

In closing, smoking is terrible for the human body. To prevent long-term smoking as an adult, it's important to talk to our children in order to prevent the initiation of this terrible habit. For those who already smoke, quitting may be a tough road, though it is possible, and the benefits far exceed the short-term difficulties. There are multiple methods to help you throughout the process. Please speak to your doctor and have a plan in place to best prepare for that quit date when it finally comes.

QUICK HITS

- Simply put, smoking is foolish. It is poison and only has negative health effects.
- NO AMOUNT IS SAFE. Even less than 1 cigarette per day substantially increases your risk of lung cancer and death.
- Quitting the habit of smoking is beneficial at any age.
- Find motivation to quit anywhere and everywhere.
- Plan ahead, speak to your physician and get others involved when you are ready to quit.
- It is okay to fail; just try again.
- E-cigarettes have their own health risks, and the long-term effects are not yet known. Importantly, vaping increases the chances of traditional smoking in teens.

Marijuana in Modern Culture

Since the early 1990s, marijuana use has steadily risen in the US.[81] This is mirrored by rising public opinion and political efforts favoring the legalization of marijuana. In 1996, California became the first state to pass laws related to medicinal marijuana.[81] In the years following, an increasing number of states have followed suit, and as of February 2020, 33 states and the District of Columbia had established medical marijuana laws, including 11 states legalizing recreational use.[81]

As a result, legalization created a community with vested financial interests, which created a widespread narrative that marijuana is "medicine."[82] A national survey of US adults subsequently revealed that 29% of adults believe smoking marijuana prevents health problems, while 18% believe smoking is "somewhat or completely safe."[83] Movies, music, and social media have also glamorized marijuana use, similar to the prior glamorization of cigarettes in popular culture. In 2016, 30% of the billboards top 40 songs in the US featured positive references to marijuana.[84] Comedies such as *Harold and Kumar Go to White Castle*, *Pineapple Express*, and *This is the End* depict heavy smoking and its consequences comedically, further popularizing its use.

Celebrities also openly promote marijuana use. Kevin Smith, an actor who starred in films featuring the characters Jay and Silent Bob, famously said that smoking marijuana saved his life when he had a heart attack (more on this later). Recently, during the COVID-19 pandemic and in an interview with Jimmy Kimmel, Seth Rogan laughed when saying, "I've smoked a truly ungodly amount of weed in the time that I've been quarantined," and, "Thank God it has been declared an essential service."[85] And as we hear more voices promoting its use, public opinion too is increasingly favorable. According to the Pew Research Center, two-thirds of Americans say the use of marijuana should be legal,[86] and with it, a growing number of major political figures support federal legalization.

This is not a political statement supporting nor opposing legalization. This is merely an effort to educate the reader on the true health effects of marijuana use, both positive and negative. Today, the view of health effects is skewed and one-sided, favoring the supposed benefits and ignoring the risks. Medically supervised use of cannabis, for example, among cancer patients is then conflated with recreational use among healthy teens.

As mentioned earlier, I juxtapose this trend with cigarettes. Just like marijuana, cigarettes were glamorized and promoted in the early twentieth century in print, in film, and on TV. The rate of smoking skyrocketed while the health effects were mostly unknown. It wasn't until 1964 that the first Surgeon General's report exposed the harmful effects of cigarette smoking.[23]

I would also compare this pattern to the use of alcohol. In 1933, Congress passed the Twenty-First Amendment, which repealed the Eighteenth Amendment.[87] This action ended prohibition and again legalized alcohol. This did not make alcohol safe. There are over 20,000 annual deaths in the US from alcoholic liver disease alone.[88] Add other health effects, as well as related car accidents and homicides, and you get a staggering death count, which we'll discuss in more detail later.

Again, this book is not intended as a political platform. My goal is to ensure that one makes and educated decision prior to smoking marijuana. Each individual should know the potential benefits and risks of use. What that person does with the information is up to them.

The Health Effects of Marijuana

The study of marijuana and its components has encountered barriers impeding the advancement of research. The US Drug Enforcement Agency (DEA) classifies it as a Schedule 1 substance; thus regulations have led to gaps in research of the health effects of cannabis products, research which is key to addressing public health questions.[89] Medical and scientific communities support efforts to allow research evaluating the safety and effectiveness of medical marijuana and its derived compounds, in order to answer the questions related to their potential medical properties.

Marijuana is a plant species within the genus Cannabis, with complex biochemical interactions in the human body. Cannabis has over 400 chemical entities, 60 of them in the family of cannabinoids, with two major compounds being THC and CBD.[90] There are specific bindings sites for cannabinoids in the brain termed the cannabinoid receptor system. These two types of receptors are called the cannabinoid receptors (CBR): CB1R and CB2R.[90] Our bodies also naturally produce cannabinoid-like chemicals, which bind to a distinct set of receptors called the endocannabinoid system.[90] CB1Rs are located mainly in the brain, but are also found in the nerves, liver, thyroid, bones, and testicular tissue. CBR2s are mostly found in the immune cells, spleen and gastrointestinal system, and to a lesser extent, the brain and nerves.[90] We found both in the placenta.

In the brain, CB1Rs mostly control inhibitory action of multiple chemical neurotransmitters, affecting functions such as cognition, memory, motor movement, and pain perception.[90] The endocannabinoids appear to maintain a balance and prevent excessive neuronal activity.[90] THC partially binds to and promotes the activation of the CB1R, creating subsequent effects that are not always straightforward due to complex interactions of multiple neurotransmitter systems.[90] CBD may weakly bind[91,90] to CB1R and CB2R, though the mechanism of action is not yet clear. Other non-cannabinoid receptors have been found, and knowledge of their biology is incomplete.[90] Lab, animal, and human data also point to potential clinical effects of THC and CBD.

A Spectrum from Good to Bad

Let's start with the good by evaluating the clinical benefits of cannabis-related products according to the National Academies of Science, Engineering, and Medicine;[92] the American Academy of Neurology;[93] the *Journal of the American Academy of Pediatrics*;[94] and the *Journal of the American Medical Association*.[95] The FDA has approved a CBD oral solution to treat seizures related to two rare and severe epilepsy disorders, termed Dravet Syndrome and Lennox-Gastaut Syndrome.[96] There is evidence that cannabis or cannabinoids reduces pain symptoms, especially in chronic nerve[93] and cancer pain.[92,95] There is evidence that oral cannabinoids are effective in reducing chemotherapy induced nausea and vomiting in adults and children.[92,95,94] In adults with multiple sclerosis, certain oral cannabinoids improved reported muscle spasms.[92,93,95] There is also evidence that oral THC (dronabinol) and marijuana may help increase weight, and possibly increase appetite, in adults with HIV.[95] There was low-quality evidence suggesting cannabinoids were associated with improvements in sleep disorders.[95] There is also very low-quality evidence for an improvement in public speaking anxiety.[95] THC capsules might be associated with improvement in tic severity in patients with Tourette syndrome.[95]

Let's continue with the 'indifferent' findings. There is no clinical evidence that cannabis nor cannabinoids lessen the risk of cancer. On the contrary, there is evidence of increased risk of testicular cancer.[92] There is insufficient data to reach a conclusion regarding the effect of cannabis on the human immune system.[92] There is no clear reduction in eye pressures in patients with glaucoma who use cannabinoids; [95] thus, the American Academy of Ophthalmology does not recommend cannabis to treat glaucoma.[97] Evidence is inconclusive to date regarding the effectiveness of medical cannabis for the management of Parkinson's disease,[93,98] although there is interest in this field given positive findings in patient surveys[99] and biologic interactions between CBD and the brain pathways affected in Parkinson's. Inhaled vaporized cannabis is being studied at the University of California at San Diego for the acute treatment of migraines, and findings are not yet available.

Let's end with the bad. There is evidence suggesting that smoking cannabis may be associated with heart attacks.[92] This makes sense given the underlying mechanisms of combustion and their relation to plaque buildup. As stated earlier, Kevin Smith said marijuana saved his life when he had a heart attack. There is a phenomenon in our body called ischemic preconditioning. The phenomenon conditions our tissues (heart in this case) to low levels of oxygen, so it can better tolerate prolonged periods without oxygen. You can do this by endurance exercise, though it may occur in a subtle form when you smoke, because the toxic smoke leads to reduced oxygen delivery. The rationale is that his marijuana smoking may have allowed his heart to better tolerate his blocked artery until doctors opened it, though it likely played a significant part in the development of the plaque that caused his heart attack in the first place. When smoked regularly, cannabis is associated with increased chronic bronchitis and respiratory symptoms, though it is unclear yet if there is a significant association with COPD, asthma, or lung cancer.[92] Based on the mechanisms of combustion and the toxic, cancer-causing chemicals it produces, it would not be unexpected for this relation to be made in the future.

It is likely that the most profound effect relates to the mental, psychological, and social effects. Cannabis use substantially increases the risk of developing schizophrenia and other psychotic disorders.[92,94] Substantial data shows a temporal association with cannabis use and future psychosis, even when correcting for many other factors associated with psychosis. In general, cannabis use leads to more than doubling the risk of future schizophrenia or similar disorders.[100] The risk is worse the younger the age and the more frequent the usage. Daily use more than triples the odds of psychotic disorders, and use of higher potency THC types increases the odds nearly five-fold.[101] There are also significant mood consequences, such as increased social anxiety and depression.[92] More frequent users are more likely to have suicidal thoughts[94] and have poorly controlled bipolar disorder.[92]

For adolescents who already have underlying mood disorders, the risk of negative behaviors is substantially higher for cannabis users compared to non-users. In fact, the risk of death by any cause was found to be 59% higher, death by overdose (of any substance) more than double, and the risk of self-harm and homicide more than triple that of non-users.[102] Even without underlying psychologic disorders, cannabis use when young is associated with more depression and suicidal behaviors later in life. The odds of a cannabis user developing depression as a young adult are 37% higher compared to a non-user.[103] What's worse, the odds of suicidal thoughts are 50% higher, and actual suicide attempts are over three times as high.[103] These poor outcomes may be because of the clouded thinking, poor judgment, and impulsivity that comes with cannabis use, especially with higher potency THC content.

There are significant cognitive consequences as well, such as impairments in learning, memory, attention, and lower-than-expected IQ scores.[92,94] This morphs into social consequences. Evidence associates cannabis use with impairments in academic achievement, education level, and social relationships, along with resultant increased rates of unemployment and low income.[92,94] The common phrase "gateway drug" also seems to apply to marijuana. There is evidence linking cannabis use and the development of substance abuse disorder for other substances, including alcohol, tobacco, and other illicit drugs.[92,94]

Is Marijuana Actually Medicinal?

Marijuana is *not* a medicine, just like the mold *Penicillium Rubens* is not medicine. We don't smoke the mold to combat bacterial infections; instead, we separate the penicillin product from the mold and then purify it for use as an antibiotic.[104] Similarly, we need to separate the CBD and THC, then purify and concentrate it for potential use in specific medical conditions. There is no FDA approved medication to date, which is delivered by means of smoking. We have plenty of aerosolized prescription drugs that we inhale as inhalers (dry powder, metered dose, or soft mist) and nebulizers, but none that we light and smoke. Marijuana is not the exception. Using combustion as the means of delivering a medication is not on a par with medical standards.

As discussed, CBD is already approved for two specific epilepsy syndromes, and there appears to be evidence supporting cannabinoids to treat pain, spasticity, nausea, vomiting and weight gain. There is interest in its potential use in Parkinson's disease. There is no clinical evidence that cannabis decreases the risk of cancer, improves the immune system, nor benefits patients with glaucoma.

However, it is important is to emphasize that cannabis use involves risks, especially in the cognitive, psychological, and social domains. This risk is especially high in the developing brains of children and adolescents, though it is also present in adults, especially with frequent use of more potent marijuana. This is in line with my professional experience working in an inpatient psychiatric unit, where every single adolescent I saw with schizophrenia, or with another psychotic disorder, had a history of marijuana use. EVERY SINGLE ONE. There also appear to be cardiovascular and pulmonary risks, though this connection is not as solid as the above. Given that smoking requires combustion, I'm confident that evidence showing cardiovascular risks, cancer risk (especially in the mouth, trachea, and lung) and other pulmonary diseases will eventually come to light. It took decades for the medical community to realize the risks of commercial cigarettes, and I expect this pattern will be the same for marijuana.

Summary: An Opinion on Marijuana

The risks of cigarettes are widely and actively circulated, plastered on the side of cigarette packs in plain sight for the purchaser. This should be the same for marijuana. This is not a statement arguing against the trend of legalization per se, but a statement emphasizing that there are obvious dangers that should be presented rather than concealed. It is up to the purchaser to decide if they wish to smoke, and I believe it should be up to local governments to decrease risk of second-hand exposure or adolescent use, just as for cigarettes.

The reality is, smoking marijuana is mostly for recreation, not for medicinal purposes. Most adults will not develop the aforementioned issues, assuming that their habit is only occasional. I emphasize "occasional" and "most adults."

The frontal lobes, responsible for impulse control, planning, working memory, and more, may not be fully developed until a person's mid-twenties.[105] Thus, I am firmly against early use and would advise any parent to educate their children about the risks of marijuana to the developing brain. I would also advise any adult with a family history of psychotic disorders or a personal history of mood disorders against this habit.

With this, I'll make a final statement in agreement with the author Alex Berenson: "Only adults — preferably over 25 — should use cannabis. And they should use only if they are psychiatrically healthy."[82] I would add that use should be only occasional and with lower THC content. Finally, if someone's reaction to smoking is paranoia and psychosis, they should avoid it altogether, as it may predispose them to psychiatric complications.

QUICK HITS

- Smoking marijuana is not "healthy."
- Chemicals in marijuana, when isolated and concentrated in medication, appear to have a specific set of medicinal properties.
- Excess marijuana has many negative health effects, the most pronounced being cognitive and psychological.
- No child or teen should smoke marijuana.
- Occasional use by an adult more than 25 years of age, who smokes marijuana with low THC content, and has no personal or family history of psychiatric disorders, is unlikely to result in major negative health risks.

3. DRINK ONLY IN MODERATION

"Wine is sunlight, held together by water."
- Galileo Galilei

Alcohol: A Brief History

Alcohol is a staple in both the modern-day America and in other, older cultures. From the ancient beer brewers in Egypt, to the wine parties of ancient Greece, to the sophisticated winery businesses of ancient Rome, alcohol has been an important aspect of life throughout human history. Even in the Bible, the first account of a public miracle performed by Jesus Of Nazareth was the turning of water into wine (John 2:1-12).[106] Historically, alcohol has been a major part of human civilization. Today, the production, sale and consumption of alcohol is a massive global industry valued at 1.4 trillion dollars in 2017. [107] The same year, US tax revenue from alcohol alone amounted to 10 billion dollars.[108]

Yet only a century earlier, in 1917, the US Congress passed the Eighteenth Amendment, which banned the making, transportation, and sale of alcohol.[109] The driving force behind this was a movement which saw alcohol as a destructive and unethical force. What followed was a bloody black market, with a rise in violent and powerful crime organizations. The Chicago mob boss, Al Capone, made as much as 100 million dollars annually,[110] which would be the equivalent of nearly 1.5 billion dollars in 2020. Crime families throughout the country gained power and wealth, leading to a rise in gang violence. In the 1920s and early 1930s, over 1,000 people were killed in New York City alone in relation to mob violence.[110]

With a change in public sentiment, a sunken economy because of the Great Depression, and a desire to create jobs and revenue, the Eighteenth Amendment was repealed in 1933, marking an end to the Prohibition Era.[109] Although today we no longer have gang wars and killings to control the sale and distribution of alcohol, the harm to people and the deaths from the effects of alcohol are higher than ever would have been expected in the 1930s.

Alcohol's Impact on Health

The alcohol we consume functions in the human body in specific ways. It's common knowledge that one can get inebriated and intoxicated from having too many drinks. This occurs through the depressant effect of ethanol, which reduces natural inhibitory signals in the brain, leading to changes associated with drunkenness (decreased attention, memory, mood changes, and drowsiness).[111] In excessive amounts, the depressant effects result in amnesia, loss of sensation, and in severe cases, decreased breathing and death.[111] This is acute alcohol poisoning, and it kills about 2,200 Americans annually.[112]

The other commonly known side effect is liver disease, which has a spectrum of injury from fatty changes (steatosis) to liver scarring (cirrhosis) and eventually liver failure.[113] Alcoholic liver disease was responsible for the deaths of over 24,000 Americans in 2019.[88] The liver sustains the greatest degree of tissue injury from heavy drinking because it is the primary site of ethanol metabolism,[113] but alcohol also causes injury and side effects far beyond the liver.

A broad range of injury and resultant diseases occurs because of excessive alcohol use. Twenty-five chronic diseases are entirely attributable to alcohol, and over 200 others are caused in part by alcohol.[114] Although not an exhaustive list, alcohol directly causes behavioral disorders, brain shrinkage (atrophy), nerve damage (neuropathy), muscle damage (myopathy), heart weakness (cardiomyopathy), stomach inflammation (gastritis), liver disease (as above), pancreas inflammation (pancreatitis) and newborn congenital abnormalities (fetal alcohol syndrome).[114] Alcohol also increases the risk of mental and behavioral disorders such as depression, neurologic conditions such as epilepsy and dementia, cardiovascular diseases such as elevated blood pressure, and many cancers, including cancer of the mouth, esophagus, stomach, liver, colon, rectum, breast, and prostate.[114] Additionally, the poor choices made while drinking can lead to significant injury and death. In young adults, the leading cause of death is unintentional injury (such as car crashes, falls, and drowning) followed by suicide and homicide.[115] It is estimated that about 30% of unintentional non-traffic related deaths, and nearly 40% of traffic deaths in the US are alcohol-related.[116] About 22% of suicide victims are legally intoxicated at the time of death.[117] Lastly, a staggering 40% of convicted murderers use alcohol before or during the crime,[118] and 40% of homicide victims had a positive blood alcohol level.[119]

Clearly, excess alcohol consumption, acutely and chronically, is detrimental to an individual and to society. Alcohol related deaths in the US have increased over the last decade,[120] and now, including all factors we've discussed so far, causes over 95,000 deaths per year in the US,[121] making it one of the leading causes of preventable death.[122]

My typical experience as a neurologist involves the treatment of chronic alcoholics in the ICU, patients with cirrhosis and yellow skin (jaundice) who are breathing through a ventilator, bleeding from the gut (which comes out the mouth and anus), swollen throughout (especially the abdomen and legs), dependent on a machine to clean their blood, with a swollen brain from the accumulation of toxic chemicals that the liver cannot process, in a coma, and desperately awaiting a transplant. What I see is the extreme end of the spectrum, although quality of life may be impacted drastically even prior to hospital admission. Family members of heavy drinkers are all too aware of and affected by this reality.

Is There a Safe Amount?

Most people believe they don't drink enough to have complications from alcohol. There clearly is a dose dependent range of injury: less alcohol, less injury, and more alcohol, more injury. This begs the question; how much do I need to drink to have negative consequences? It's difficult to give ranges for all the aforementioned conditions, though we know ranges that are a general predictor for more severe cases of alcoholic liver disease. These are 40 to 80 grams of ethanol per day for men and 20 to 40 grams of ethanol per day for women for more than 10 to 12 years.[113]

Let's convert that to the number of drinks consumed. A standard drink equivalent contains 14 grams of ethanol.[123] A standard drink *volume*, however, differs by beverage type. This volume is 12 fluid ounces of beer, 5 fluid ounces of wine, and 1.5 fluid ounces of hard liquor.[123] So mathematically, that equates to about 3 to 6 standard drinks per day in men, and 1½ to 3 standard drinks per day in women, consumed regularly for slightly more than a decade. That's a 6-pack of beer a day for a man and half a bottle of wine for a woman, on the high end.

We can also look at consequences for those who are not daily but weekend binge drinkers. We define binge drinking as consuming five or more drinks for men, and 4 or more drinks for women, within a two-hour span.[124] About one in six Americans binge drink four times a month (every weekend). During a binge, they typically have about seven drinks.[125] Binge drinking has similar health effects as chronic excess alcohol use, though the immediate behavioral effects are especially troublesome. In fact, of the 93,000 deaths per year in the US related to alcohol, more than half are due to binge drinking and the subsequent behavioral consequences such as car crashes, alcohol poisoning, suicide, and violence.[125]

Although there are a lot of negatives associated with alcohol, it would be inaccurate to say it's all bad. Prior observations noted that low-to-moderate alcohol consumption was associated with lower risk of heart disease; though clearly, higher consumption was associated with higher risk of certain cancers, cirrhosis, and other health effects, as noted above.[126] A large analysis, combining data from 34 studies with over 1 million study subjects, demonstrated a "J-shaped relationship" between alcohol and total mortality.[126] (An example of a J shaped relationship can be found in **Figure 5**). That is, low levels of alcohol consumption appear to be associated with reduced total deaths compared to no alcohol use, while high levels are associated with increased deaths.

Studies have also looked at alcohol levels and the relationship between various diseases. For many conditions, no amount of alcohol is beneficial. For example, for many cancers (such as of the mouth, esophagus, larynx, colon, rectum, liver, and breast), high blood pressure, pancreatitis, and liver disease,[127] there was *no* benefit at any level of alcohol use. In fact, the contrary was found: with increasing alcohol consumption came significantly increased risk of these conditions.[127]

Some diseases, though, appear to benefit from light alcohol use. Heart disease from arterial plaque buildup also appears to have a J-shape relation to alcohol consumption. At low alcohol consumption of 20 grams per day (about 1.5 drinks), there appears to be a reduction in risk of heart disease.[127] Similar to heart disease, light alcohol consumption of 12 to 24 grams per day (about one or two drinks) may protect against strokes, while heavier amounts actually increase the risk of stroke and brain bleeds.[128] Additionally, consuming a low amount of alcohol might lower the risk of developing chronic kidney disease.[129] Lastly, light alcohol consumption seems to be associated with a lower risk of diabetes.[130]

Why do we see the benefits in these conditions? It's hypothesized that, when consumed AT LOW LEVELS, alcohol may

- increase good cholesterol,
- decrease clotting through several mechanisms,
- have beneficial effects in the inner lining of blood vessels,
- decrease inflammation, and
- have a positive effect on sugar metabolism .[126,131]

The benefits, particularly regarding heart disease, are seen in wine drinkers over non-wine drinkers, suggesting that the substances present in wine may be responsible for the positive effects.[132] Other data shows that a substantial portion of the benefit is derived from the alcohol rather than other components of the beverage.[133]

Closing Opinion on Alcohol

The preceding list of possible benefits is not an endorsement to drink daily. I DO NOT recommend that you drink if you do not do so already. But if you already drink, do so lightly, up to one drink per day to keep it simple. Certain people should not drink at all, such as women who are or may be pregnant, youth, and people who take medications that interact with alcohol and recovering alcoholics.[134] There are certain health conditions (as mentioned above), where drinking should probably be avoided altogether.

Thus, I would emphasize, if you do not drink, there is no need to start. If you do drink, then do so in low amounts of no more than one drink per day, preferably wine, and at the proper serving size. I personally would not drink daily, although several days a week might have some health benefits. Cessation of light to moderate drinking will unlikely have withdrawal effects and is unlikely to cause any behavioral changes leading to dangerous decision making.

QUICK HITS

- If you do not drink, there is no need to start.
- If you already drink, limit yourself to one drink per day.
- Avoid binge drinking, defined as greater than five drinks over a two-hour span.
- Know what a drink equivalent is: 12 oz. of beer, 5 oz. of wine and 1.5 oz. of liquor.
- If you choose to drink, wine may be a healthier option than beer or liquor.
- DO NOT drink if pregnant.
- Speak to your physician if you are at higher risk because of certain medications or having health conditions.

4. PURSUE A HEALTHY WEIGHT

"Losing 10 grams of excessive fat is way more beneficial for our health than wearing something that makes us look 10 kilograms lighter."
- Mokokoma Mokhonoana

Introduction to an Epidemic

An epidemic occurring in the US has slowly affected more and more Americans over the last several decades. Now, for the first time in centuries, the current generation of children in America may have shorter life expectancies than their parents.[135] In fact, for the past thousand years, human life expectancies have seen a slow and steady increase; now, life expectancy at birth, and even for individuals at older ages, are expected to level off and even decline within the first half of this century.[136] It is not because of a virus or a contagion. A drug or a new disease is not causing this historical change. Instead, our societal habits have led to a rise in the epidemic called obesity.

Obesity by the Numbers

Obesity is defined by a ratio of weight (in kilograms) divided by height (in meters squared).[137] Simply put, weight over height.

We term this Body Mass Index (BMI). There are simple online calculators to check one's own BMI. **I invite you to search for your own BMI now prior to continuing.** In any search engine, type "What's my BMI?" and you'll have many options to instantly calculate that figure. It correlates well with body fat in most people, except for athletes who have significantly increased lean muscle mass.[138] A BMI of 25 and higher is categorized as overweight, while 30 and higher is categorized as obese (Table 1).[139,140] As an example, a person 5 feet 9 inches tall has a BMI of 30 at 203 pounds or more.[137] A BMI of 40 and higher is categorized as severe obesity. Using the example above, the same person must weigh 271 pounds or more to reach severe obesity.[137]

Currently, being overweight is more common than not. In the US, greater than 65% of adults are overweight.[141] As of 2018, 42% of Americans were obese.[142] In adults, the rate of obesity was highest amongst Blacks (50%) and lowest amongst Asians (17%).[142] In the same year, 9% of adults were severely obese, with rates even higher among women compared to men.[142] Since as recently as the year 2000, the rate of obesity has increased by 39%, while the rate of severe obesity has increased by a staggering 96%.[142] By comparison, in the early 1960s, the rate of obesity in American adults was only 13%.[143]

Childhood obesity is also an increasing concern. As of 2018, 19% of Americans younger than 19 years old were obese. The rate of obesity was highest in Hispanics (26%) and lowest in Asians (9%). By comparison, in the early 1970s, the rate of obesity in children and adolescents was only 5%. It has steadily risen since, increasing by 39% in the last 2 decades alone.[144]

As a country, we are gaining weight; we are heavier than we should be, and we know it. Polling data shows that the average American is 13 pounds heavier in 2007 compared to 1990, increasing to 17 pounds for women.[145] What's more, 68% stated their current weight was greater than their perceived goal weight by an average of 17 pounds, increasing to 21 pounds for women.[145] It's clear that as a society, we have gained weight; but we are not alone.

Worldwide, there were 650 million people categorized as obese in 2016, a value that has nearly tripled since 1975.[146] Currently, most of the world's population live in countries where complications from being overweight kill more people than the complications of being underweight.[146] As put by *The Los Angeles Times*, "a tidal wave of fat, and the ailments that come with it, now appears virtually inevitable in the United States,"[147] as data projects a continued trend in increasing obesity, resulting in nearly one in two adults being obese, and nearly one in four being severely obese by the year 2030.[148]

The question then arises: what has changed in our society that has created this public health problem? Before discussing environmental and cultural changes leading to this epidemic, we'll first put it into context by briefly discussing how we regulate our body weight.

BMI	Classification
Less than 18.5	Underweight
18.5 to 24.9	Healthy Weight
25 to 29.9	Overweight
30 or more	Obese
30 to 34.9	Class 1
35 to 39.5	Class 2
Greater than 40	Class 3 (Severe)
Greater than 50	Class 4 (Super)
Greater than 60	Class 5 (Super-Super)

Table 1: Weight category based on BMI

Regulation of Weight

Body weight is directly correlated with energy balance, which states that "when the amount of energy needed by the body is balanced with the amount consumed in the diet, weight will remain constant."[138] The energy in food can be measured in kilocalories (calories). If the energy eaten is greater than the energy burned, excess energy will be stored and result in weight gain. Excess energy is stored in different forms, fat being most important when intake far exceeds energy used. When the energy eaten in food is less than our body's energy requirements, we meet the additional need by breaking down what we have stored as glycogen, muscle, and fat.[138] Thus, fat is a backup storage unit for energy needs. It is stored efficiently, and can be stored in virtually unlimited amounts in adipose (fat) tissue.[138]

Energy use is the other critical part of this energy balance. Our total energy use is the sum of the Basal Metabolic Rate (BMR), physical activity, and the Thermic Effect of Food (TEF).[138] BMR, simply put, is the energy to maintain basic body functions like breathing and blood flow. It is proportional to lean body mass.[138] This is why men with higher levels of lean body mass have higher metabolic rates than women, and why metabolism decreases with age. In essence, BMR correlates well with muscle mass. The BMR accounts for up 60-75% of the body's total energy requirements.[138]

Physical activity is the second highest component of energy use, but this varies depending on your activity level. A professional soccer player's proportion of energy use from physical activity is much higher than that of a software engineer, who spends most of the day sitting at a desk. Strenuous exercise is not the only important component of physical activity. Minor activities like involuntary exercise (such as fidgeting, maintaining posture, and standing) may considerably alter a person's susceptibility to weight gain.[138] Lastly, the TEF is the temporary increase in energy use after eating, due to digesting, metabolizing, and storing food; it can last several hours.[138] It also accounts for approximately 10% of daily energy use,[138] though this can differ depending on what one eats.

Although energy balance is a simple concept (*energy in - energy out = net energy*), the relationship between energy balance and body fat is more complicated. Genetic and hormonal factors not only affect how our body uses energy, but affects how much body fat we accumulate. What we know is that humans are efficient at storing energy, which stems from our ancestors, who were hunters and gatherers. Like lions or bears, our ancestors had an inconsistent availability of food. They had successful and unsuccessful hunts and might go extended periods of time without food. Our ancestors used large amounts of energy in all aspects of life, from building shelters and traveling on foot, to defending themselves from animals and hunting. They needed to have efficient mechanisms to maintain weight. Today, those mechanisms that defend against weight loss are stronger than those that prevent weight gain,[138] which makes it easy to see how societal changes and decreases physical activity relate to the obesity epidemic.

Modern Habits

Today, food is relatively cheap and widely available. With rare exceptions, we don't need to burn significant amounts of energy to get food, to travel, or to find shelter.[149] Compared to just decades ago, Americans are eating bigger portions[150] and eating out more.[151] The average American ate almost 20% more calories in the year 2000 than they did in 1983.[150] The percentage of meals eaten away from home doubled between the 1970s and the 1990s.[152] With this came a rise in fast food consumption, with an average of 13% of daily calories coming from fast food between 2003 and 2006.[153] Food portion sizes in restaurants have doubled or tripled over the last 20 years.[154]

At the same time, there has been a decrease in physical activity both at work and in our leisure time. Fewer Americans work in agriculture and on factory floors, and more are sitting throughout the workday.[150] In the 1960s, nearly 50% of jobs in the US required at least moderate physical activity; today, less than 20% require this energy.[155] This translates to an average decline of about 140 calories a day in physical activity, which closely correlates to the average weight gain over a 50-year period.[155]

Outside of work, factors from technology and community design influence our sedentary behaviors.[151] The development of sprawling suburbs has led to less walking and more drive time to school and work. Television viewing, and other sedentary activities in front of screens, has become the predominant form of leisure activity.[152] Although hereditary factors are involved in energy use and weight gain, the genes within a population take generations to change.[138] However, the speed by which the obesity epidemic has gained a foothold argues against a genetic cause,[156] and supports the view that cultural factors, mainly increased food consumption and decreased physical activity, are the major contributors.

A Real Health Crises

The obesity epidemic has also become a public health crisis. Obesity is associated with many chronic health conditions and leads to excess death. In fact, between 1986 and 2006, being overweight and obese was likely responsible (the root cause) for

18% of deaths among US adults.[157] That's nearly one of every five deaths. Obesity has catapulted to become a leader in preventable death, trailing only smoking and high blood pressure as the third most common cause of death from modifiable risk factors, killing an estimated 216,000 Americans in 2005 alone.[18]

Obesity is also costly. According to the Centers for Disease Control (CDC), obesity-related medical care costs in the US were nearly 150 billion dollars in 2008.[156] The national productivity costs of obesity-related absenteeism is as high as 6 billion dollars annually.[156] Obesity is deadly because of the long list of associated health conditions, including but not limited to high blood pressure, abnormal cholesterol levels, diabetes, heart disease, stroke, gallbladder disease, osteoarthritis, sleep apnea, cognitive dysfunction, fatty liver disease, and many types of cancer.[156,158] Each of these illnesses involves potentially costly medical treatment.

High blood pressure itself is a leading cause of death because of its strong association with heart disease and strokes, and estimates suggest that 78% of primary hypertension in men, and 65% in women, can be linked to excess weight gain.[141] Obesity is a major risk factor for type 2 diabetes, and much of the increase in the rates of diabetes overall in the US is because of the increasing rates of obesity.[159] To put the risk into perspective, compared to a woman of healthy weight, an 18-year-old obese woman has a 38% higher lifetime risk of developing diabetes, increasing to 58% with Class 2 obesity.[160]

This isn't just theoretical risk analysis; it's an actual relation that's manifesting in real life. In fact, 85% of people with type 2 diabetes are overweight or obese.[159] Obesity is also associated with alterations in the metabolism of cholesterol, resulting in approximately 60-70% of patients with obesity having abnormal cholesterol levels.[161] The association of obesity with these three conditions cannot be stressed enough, because all three are intimately related to plaque buildup in arteries, which is the underlying cause of heart attacks, and a major cause of stroke — both potentially fatal. This relationship is likely why obesity is a significant risk factor for heart disease and strokes. As an example, obese men have a 65% increased risk of heart disease and an 85% increased risk of stroke compared to men of healthy weight.[162]

Obesity is also linked with many health effects that are independent of "cardiovascular risk factors." Being overweight and obese is associated with an increased risk of at least 17 different cancers including but not limited to: uterine, gallbladder, kidney, cervix, thyroid, leukemia, liver, colon, ovarian, and breast cancer.[163] These are not inconsequential cancers. Breast, ovarian, and uterine/cervical cancer make up the second, fifth, and sixth leading causes of cancer-related deaths in women, killing over 67,000 women in 2018.[12] In post-menopausal women, obesity leads to a 20 to 40% increased risk in developing breast cancer.[164] From a population perspective, if all obese and overweight women achieved a normal BMI, 16% of post-menopausal breast cancers could be prevented.[165] That amounts to 6,794 avoided deaths annually from breast cancer, based on 2018 data, by weight management alone. Obese and overweight women are also two to four times as likely to develop cancer in the inner lining of the uterus, and for every five-point increase in a woman's BMI, the risk of ovarian cancer increases by 10%.[164]

Obesity affects not only women and their specific cancers; this increased risk affects both women and men. Notably, colon cancer is the second leading cause of cancer deaths overall, killing over 52,000 Americans in 2018.[12] People who are obese are about 30% more likely to develop colorectal cancer.[164] In Europe, around 11% of colorectal cancer cases are attributed to being overweight and obese.[166] As rates of obesity in the US exceed those of Europe, this percentage is likely higher in the US. If we use Europe's percentage to extrapolate numbers (knowing the true percentage may be higher), we might have 5,737 avoided deaths per year from colon cancer in 2018 by weight management alone.

To conclude, we can elaborate on some less familiar health associations. Chronic liver disease and cirrhosis kill over 41,000 Americans annually.[167] Most immediately think of alcohol as the cause of cirrhosis, though it is *not* the leading cause of cirrhosis in the US; that unfortunate prize goes to fatty liver disease, accounting for over 50% of cases of chronic liver disease and cirrhosis.[168] It has become the most common cause of chronic liver disease because of increased obesity in our population.[169] Lastly, obesity has cognitive and psychological consequences. When compared with individuals at healthy weight, those with obesity appear to have a 34% higher risk of dementia.[170] Weight loss, in people who are overweight and obese, is associated with improved attention, memory, and overall cognitive performance.[171] As the burden of dementia in the US is expected to increase in the coming decades, the association with obesity, and the increasing rates of obesity, will have major public health consequences in dementia care and healthcare costs. As for psychological consequences, data shows increased odds of mood disorders (including major depression and mania), anxiety disorders, and personality disorders (including antisocial and avoidant) in obese and severely obese people compared to those at healthy weight.[172] The association between obesity and depression has also been repeatedly showed. It is estimated that people who are obese have a 55% increased risk of depression.[173] The association is stronger in woman than in men. In women, there is even an increased risk of suicidal thoughts.[174]

The obesity epidemic is clearly having negative health consequences for individuals and for the population. The higher a person's BMI category is, the more risk there is of potential deadly medical complications in the future (Figure 5).[175] Individually, someone who is obese may pass a "standard health check" at a single point in time. They may have normal blood pressure and sugar levels and be considered healthy. But like smoking, it takes time to develop the associated downstream medical complications. But over time, one is continually exposed to increased risk of a variety of negative health consequences. We can't change age, we can't change genetics, but we *can* change unhealthy weight and lessen our health risks, even in the face of current cultural trends that ignore these very real medical truths.

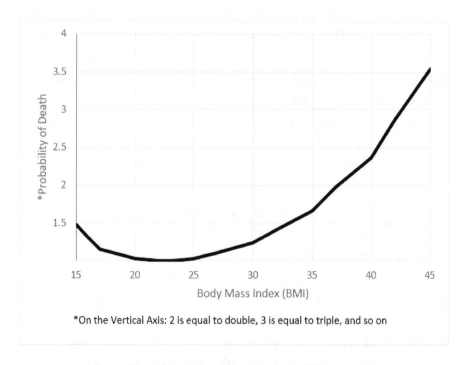

*On the Vertical Axis: 2 is equal to double, 3 is equal to triple, and so on

Figure 5: Risk of Death based on BMI Categories

Healthy Body or Body Positivity

Today, we are seeing a cultural movement of body positivity. The premise of the movement is wonderful! The idea of self-confidence, of loving and appreciating oneself while accepting the flaws **we all have,** is an important lesson. Developing a positive image of oneself today is especially important given the vile content on social media, the relentless bullying that can occur in schools and workplaces, and the constant exposure to "influencers" with unrealistic body standards.

In our society, the cultural pendulum swings rather precipitously. In 2020, the musician Adele made headlines in the news after losing about 100 pounds[176] to be a healthy mom for her children. The physical transformation also had positive psychological effects, as it is quoted that "she is more confident, dresses differently and she just seems happier overall."[177] While many had supportive messages for her, there was also an abundance of negative opinions about her weight loss, especially attacking the positive remarks made to her about looking "beautiful."

This aggressiveness towards promoting weight loss was much clearer after fitness celebrity Jillian Michaels made comments regarding body positivity messages from celebrities like Lizzo and plus-size model Ashley Graham. She stated: "Why are we celebrating her [Lizzo's] body? Why does it matter? Why aren't we celebrating her music? 'Cause it isn't going to be awesome if she gets diabetes."[178] Michaels received harsh criticism online and on social media, claiming she was "fat phobic" and was "body shaming" Lizzo.[178] Though she clearly could have been more tactful, the message was not incorrect. There are undeniable health risks associated with obesity; therefore, celebrating obesity while being blind to these risks is not the optimum approach to body positivity. Promoting the idea that any body shape is beautiful and feeling empowered by one's own size should not be done at the expense of recognizing current or future health risks.

A perfect example was the recent *Cosmopolitan* magazine cover (February 2021) featuring women who were obese with the title "This is Healthy."[179] I understand the desire to be inclusive of people of all shapes and sizes. I applaud the effort to support people who may feel harassed and "fat shamed" simply for being obese. But I also vehemently disagree with lying about the health risks. **Obesity is not healthy**, period. Why not title the cover "This is Beautiful" to promote body positivity without also misleading readers?

Would *Cosmopolitan*, or any other magazine, do a cover shoot showing someone smoking a cigarette, with the caption stating, "This is healthy?" I doubt it. Nobody argues that smoking is healthy, or that by making assumptions about future health risks, we stigmatize smokers. On the contrary, we actively advertise the dangers of smoking based on assumed future risks, even if a smoker is healthy *at the moment*.

Obesity trails only smoking and high blood pressure as a leading cause of death from modifiable risk factors. So, let's not proclaim being overweight as healthy. It is without debate that obesity is a significant risk factor for many conditions, including premature death. Therefore, we can promote self-confidence and acceptance in one's body while also honestly promoting normal (healthy) weight for health and wellbeing.

A Personal Opinion

So, what to do? What am I advocating? For one, let us all recognize that there is always room for self-improvement. We are imperfect beings, and there is no harm in recognizing that.

Also, weight can fluctuate during our lives for many reasons. If we are overweight or obese, it is okay to be proactive about it and to lose weight to improve our health. This does not make a person "fat phobic," and it should not make you feel that losing weight is only about vanity. It is not. It is about seeking better health.

The goal is to achieve a healthy weight, not an idealized figure. This is true for both young and old, because age is not a barrier to successful weight loss. Lifestyle programs have been similarly effective at promoting weight loss and lowering BMI in younger and older adults.[180] I will only briefly touch on the lifestyle modifications here, as I will discuss this in detail in the following chapters.

As stated before, energy balance and body weight result from a simple relation between calories consumed versus calories burned. When one consumes more calories than they burn, they gain weight. It just so happens to be much easier to consume calories than it is to burn them. That's an inescapable reality. As an example, the most commonly ordered drink at Starbucks by college students in the Northeastern US is the White Mocha Frappuccino;[181] the Grande (16 oz.) size contains 410 calories.[182] To burn an equal amount of calories, a 160-pound person would have to run three miles at a pace of 13 minutes per mile.[183] Can we agree it is much easier to drink one less White Mocha than it is to run three miles?

I am often told by patients with obesity that they eat well and try to be active, but still gain weight. I never doubt that a genuine effort is being made; however, available literature shows that individuals who are obese significantly under report food intake.[138,184] If burned calories are greater than consumed calories, one will lose weight. The following chapters will go into detail on healthy eating and physical activity. For now, I'll touch on some applicable "cheat codes" or "life hacks" that may help shift the energy balance equation in favor of healthy weight management.

Life Hacks for Weight Management

Since the energy balance equation is more easily adjusted by reducing calories consumed than by increasing calories burned, we will first address simple tricks to adjust intake, which, over time, can account for significant weight loss. Additional "hacks" to increase energy use will immediately follow.

Decreasing Calories Consumed

1. **Replace sugar-sweetened drinks (such as soda and juice) with water**. On average, US adults consume 145 calories per day from sweetened drinks.[185] If this is replaced by water just five days a week, it would equal 10 pounds worth of excess calories avoided per year.

2. **Drink low-fat, low-sugar coffee options**. In the US, about 30 million American adults drink specialty coffee (such as mochas and lattes) beverages daily.[186] A Grande White Mocha, with whole milk and whip cream, is 410 calories. If 2% milk is used instead, and we exclude whip cream, the calorie count decreases to 290 — a 120-calorie difference. If replaced only three days out of the week, it could equal about 5 pounds of excess calories avoided per year.

3. **Be mindful when using salad dressing**. About one out of five Americans eat salad on any given day.[187] Of these salads, 86% have salad dressing.[187] Deceptively high calorie counts in dressings can foil attempts to be healthy when eating salad. On

average, dressings account for over 100 calories per salad serving;[187] though creamy dressings like blue cheese, ranch, and Thousand Island may be higher. Consider healthy alternatives like lemon, vinegar, and olive oil combined with your favorite seasonings, or use less by ordering the dressing on the side to control the portion.

4. **Avoid overeating**. This is a broad statement and less of a trick, though a few simple tips may help decrease appetite and result in portion control during a meal.

Drink water before your meal. Doing so helps decrease the amount of food needed to fill the stomach to activate stretch receptors and cause a feeling of fullness. In one study, drinking 500 ml (~ 2 cups) of water 30 minutes before a meal led to a 13% reduction in calorie intake.[188]

Chew your food thoroughly. The more one chews, the longer it takes to eat a meal, and the more time the body has to signal the sensation of fullness, which makes it a potential behavioral strategy to reduce calorie intake. Chewing food twice as long as usual decreased food intake by 15% according to one study.[189]

Chew gum at the end of a meal. The sense of fullness signals us to stop eating. In one study, rates of fullness after chewing gum for five minutes was 17% higher compared to not chewing gum, increasing to 35% after 30 minutes.[190]

Use smaller plates. The dinner plate size in the US is increasing. In the 1980s, the typical diameter of a dinner plate was 25 cm, and in the 2000s it was 30 cm.[191] This increase in diameter results in an increase in total area of 44%. Larger plates influence the perception of food portion size[192] and are linked to larger portions and greater caloric intake. One study using buffet diners found that those with larger plates ate 45% more food than those with smaller plates.[193]

5. Decrease alcohol intake. Carbohydrates and proteins have four calories per gram, while alcohol has seven calories per gram. Calories from alcohol are "empty calories" as they have no nutritional value. Besides being a source of calories, alcohol affects our natural mechanisms of metabolism, in part, by suppressing fat oxidation, suppressing muscle building[194] and altering hormones, which can lead to excess energy balance and weight gain.[195]

6. Adjust food ratios. We'll go into much more detail on recommended nutrition later in this book, but briefly, most Americans don't get enough fruits and vegetables. This leads to an easy target and health priority for a life hack. A good way to get more vegetables in one's diet while decreasing calories consumed is to first fill half your plate with fruits and/or vegetables. That automatically leaves less space for high-calorie foods and leads to decreased energy intake while also getting the healthy vegetables we lack.

7. **Keep a food diary**. A more time-consuming, but effective means of managing food intake is being consciously aware of how much and what you are eating. One can do this by keeping a food diary. Because we know that many under report the amount of food they eat, a food diary helps bridge a gap between perception and reality. The Weight Loss Maintenance Trial Research group found that those who kept food records six days a week, documenting everything they ate and drank on those days, lost about twice the weight as those who kept food records one day a week or less.[196]

Increasing Calories Burned

1. **Only use the stairs**. I call this the staircase challenge. In 2018, 108.5 million Americans rented their homes.[197] Of these renters, 37% (over 40 million) lived in apartments.[198] Add to this number

apartment owners and people who work in multistory buildings, and you have a large section of the population that has easy access to stairs. On average, a person burns 0.17 calories for every step climbed and 0.05 calories per step descended.[199] The result: if a person takes the stairs for just five stories per day instead of using the elevator, that would equal to about seven to eight lbs. lost in five years. That's doesn't seem like a lot, but to put into context, the average American man weights 184 lbs. in his twenties and 200 lbs. in his thirties.[200] This one simple habit could offset the gradual weight gain that most adults experience.

2. **Park farther away**. US drivers spend an average of 17 hours a year searching for parking spots.[201] We tend to search for the closest, most convenient spot to park. The overall impact of adding 100 to 200 feet of walking distance to go shopping is small, but it can help with changing habits and lead to a less sedentary lifestyle. The more steps walked over time, the more calories burned, and the easier it becomes to achieve a balance in the energy equation.

3. **Increase standing time**. Excess sitting time is linked to obesity, heart disease, cancer, diabetes, and death.[202] The average American adult sits six to seven hours a day, and a quarter of adults sit over eight hours per day.[202] Increasing standing time at work or home is an easy way to change our energy use and mitigate the above risks. When we stand, we activate muscles required to maintain posture. This alone uses energy and burns more calories than sitting. On average, a man who weighs 160 pounds will burn about 40 calories more per hour when standing compared to sitting.[203] Standing for just one extra hour a day would be the equivalent of about four pounds per year, offsetting gradual weight gain.

This list of easy-to-apply behavior modifications can lead to reduced calorie intake and increased energy use. Perhaps successful application of some of these can be a steppingstone to a change in overall habits. As you can see, there aren't many secrets to burning more calories; one just has to be more active. These tips increase energy use within an existing routine. As we'll see in the next chapter, anything more will require an additional commitment of effort and time. I do not believe in "fad" diets. Instead, I support a slow approach, where one's perception of what makes up a meal evolves over time, inherently leading to a modification of what and how much one eats; eventually, the new approach becomes second nature. This intake, along with changes in physical activity to where we innately desire movement and become less sedentary, can lead to healthy weight and to overall benefits in physical abilities and mental health.

QUICK HITS

- Obesity has very real and serious adverse health consequences.
- Promoting weight loss for the improvement of health is not "fat phobia."
- The goal is to achieve a healthy weight, not an idealized figure.
- Energy balance is simply calories consumed minus calories burned.
- Work on decreasing calories consumed and increasing calories burned over time. It will take effort and behavioral change, but with time, it can be accomplished.

5. INCREASE PHYSICAL ACTIVITY

"Exercise should be regarded as tribute to the heart."
- Gene Tunney

Introduction to Fitness

In our society, the term "fitness" is often associated with physique. The covers of fitness magazines around the country feature muscular athletes with chiseled bodies appearing like the statues of Greek gods. Through exercise, we can change our body composition and more closely achieve our own personal physique goals, though more importantly, exercising to improve fitness comes with many health benefits. Here, we'll focus on those benefits.

The correlation between fitness and health has been long known, predating modern medicine by thousands of years. From ancient civilizations in India and China in the East, to Greece and Rome in the West, exercise has been viewed as a form of medicine.[204] In India, between 700 and 100 BC, a physician named Susruta described exercise as being "absolutely conducive to a better preservation of health".[204] In China, from around 25 BC to 250 AD, Hua Tuo advocated for exercise because of its yang (or energizing) effect.[204] Between about 460 and 370 BC, the Greek physician Hippocrates, considered the father of scientific medicine, wrote that "eating alone will not keep a man well, he must also take exercise." He also believed that idleness (inactivity) and overpowering food consumptions (overeating) could lead to disease.[204] In ancient Rome, the most important physician of his time, Gladius Galenus, advocated for the use of exercise in medicine, influencing the overall practice of medicine throughout the Arab and European regions for more than a thousand years.[204] Like the physicians of old, the physicians of today know very well that there are many health benefits associated with exercise and fitness. But fitness is a very broad, overarching term. We can break it down into components to better understand how being fit and exercising to achieve fitness also leads to improved health.

Depending on the source, we can break fitness down to as many as 11 separate components, though I will hone these down to four parts: endurance, strength, flexibility, and balance. Other components, like reaction time, speed, and coordination, are more related to athletic prowess. Endurance is achieved by aerobic exercise through activities such as swimming, jogging, or cycling. Strength is developed through resistance exercise via activities like pushups, pullups, and weightlifting. Flexibility and balance are developed through activities involving stretching and movement. Each has independent and overlapping health benefits; that together, they lead to better health outcomes.

Endurance and Health

Aerobic exercise is the primary form of physical activity discussed when evaluating health outcomes. An abundance of data shows its benefits to physical, mental, and emotional health. As emphasized earlier, the leading causes of death worldwide are heart disease and stroke. In the US, heart disease is the leader, while stroke is the fifth leading cause. Both entities are driven by risk factors such as abnormal cholesterol levels, diabetes, and elevated blood pressure. All can be altered by physical activity.

Aerobic exercise has broad beneficial effects on cholesterol levels.[205] It also has beneficial effects on blood sugar control. In fact, it is associated with decreased insulin resistance, lower risk of developing diabetes,[206] improved long-term blood sugar levels, and lower risk of dying for people with type 1 and type 2 diabetes.[207] It can also improve blood pressure.[208] Studies have found reductions in blood pressure with as little as 30 minutes of aerobic exercise, 3 times a week.[209] High blood pressure, diabetes and abnormal cholesterol are intricately related to arterial plaque development, which is itself associated with stroke and heart disease. Aerobic exercise has positive effects on each of these three risk factors, thus indirectly decreasing the risk of stroke and heart disease. What's more, it directly impacts the biochemical makeup of blood vessel walls, which slows progression of plaque development.[208] Exercising just 3.5 hours a week can stop the progression of arterial plaques in the heart after a year.[210] With five hours, there can be an actual regression of plaques.[210] So, directly and indirectly, exercise results in improved heart disease and stroke outcomes. Findings suggest that regular moderate aerobic exercise reduces the risk of stroke by 18-20% and the risk of heart disease by 15-22% in men and women.[211] The reductions are even higher with high-intensity exercise.[211]

In addition to cardiovascular health benefits, aerobic exercise is also linked to reduced risk of cancers involving the bladder, breast, colon, endometrium, esophagus, kidney, and stomach with some evidence linking it to lower lung cancer risk.[206,212] Given that cancer is the second leading cause of death and a leading cause of disability in the US, I cannot overstate the importance of this simple behavioral modification. Lung cancer is the leading cause of cancer deaths in the US, and there is some evidence that aerobic exercise is associated with reduced lung cancer risk, though differences in smoking habits may confound that association.[212] The data, though, suggests that with high amounts of exercise, the risk of lung cancer is reduced in smokers by 20% and in former smokers by 32%.[213] Colon cancer is the second leading cause of cancer death in the US. High amounts of exercise may result in a 19% lower risk of developing colon cancer compared to being physically inactive.[212] Breast cancer is the fourth leading cause of cancer-related deaths in the US. Women who do high amounts of exercise may have a 12% lower risk of breast cancer compared to women who are physically inactive.[214] The reduction is more robust (22%) in women who have never used hormone replacement therapy.[214] The risk of the other cancers listed above appears to be reduced by approximately 10% to 20% with high exercise levels.[215] Finally, besides having a decreased risk of developing cancer, research has found that aerobic exercise may improve survival in patients with established cancers. Data suggests that with high amounts of exercise, patients with breast cancer may have a 40% lower risk of death from breast cancer, those with colon cancer may have a 30% lower risk of death from colon cancer, and those with prostate cancer may have a 33% lower risk of death from prostate cancer.[212]

As stated above, regular aerobic exercise also has mental health benefits. In older individuals who already have cognitive decline, just 45 minutes of exercise, three times a week, appears to improve "executive functioning" in as little as six months.[216] Executive functioning includes processes like attention, planning, problem solving, working memory, abstract thinking, self-control, emotional regulation, decision making, and more.[217] The above data also showed that after six months, "cognitive age" improved by 8.8 years.[216] These benefits extend to young, otherwise healthy people as well. Aerobic exercise for just 30 minutes a day, 4 days a week, improves executive functioning and (impressively so) can increase the thickness of the outer layer of the brain.[218] Long-term data has shown that exercising in our forties, as little as twice a week, may reduce the risk of developing dementia later in life.[219,220] These positive effects are not restricted to adults; children, too, have improved performance on academic achievement tests, executive functioning, processing speed, and memory with physical activity.[206] These findings show that being physically active, particularly through aerobic exercise, is beneficial for brain health at any age, can improve cognitive functioning, and may reduce the risk of dementia.[206]

Lastly, exercise has psychological benefits that lead to improved emotional health. In 2017, over 17 million US adults suffered from major depression, representing 7.1% of all US adults.[221] In the past decade, the percentage of adults with depression did not significantly change,[222] though for adolescents, it increased by 8%,[223] affecting 3.2 million teens.[221] Depression especially affects teenage girls, with a staggering one in five teenage girls having suffered from major depression in 2017.[221] The benefits of aerobic exercise for depressive symptoms are extensive. Data suggests that just 35 minutes of daily exercise may help reduce the risk of developing major depression by 17%, even in individuals with high genetic risk of depression.[224,225] In patients with established major depressive disorder, aerobic exercise for 45 minutes a day, three days a week, has shown significant antidepressant effects,[226] which may be as equally effective as antidepressant medical treatments.[227] Depression and anxiety commonly occur together. Exercise also appears to reduce short-term feelings of anxiety and long-term anxiety in people with and without established anxiety disorders.[206] Finally, aerobic activity is associated with improved sleep outcomes, including increased efficiency, quality, and less daytime sleepiness.[206] Given that long-term sleep loss is linked with obesity, diabetes, high blood pressure, heart disease, anxiety, depression and more, improving the efficiency and quality of sleep is an integral part of our overall improvement in health.

Strength and Health

Exercise, mostly studied as aerobic activity, clearly has an abundance of health benefits. But as stated previously, fitness includes multiple components, with aerobic fitness representing only one aspect of the whole. Let's talk now about the other core aspects of fitness and how they result in improved health.

Resistance exercise for strength is most known for its effects on increasing muscle mass, but it has many other health benefits that are less commonly known. Starting with the basics, increased strength improves one's ability to perform daily functional activities, from simple tasks like lifting grocery bags to harder tasks like moving a couch to vacuum. When young, we may take these activities for granted, though as we age, the ability to remain physically independent becomes a treasure, difficult to let go and important to our mental health. Other benefits related to our mental health include improvements in one's own body image, perceived physical appearance (even more so than with aerobic activity),[228] and decreased levels of anxiety.[229] Resistance exercise has also been shown to improve cognitive functioning, with benefits more pronounced than "cognitive training."[230]

The physical benefits of resistance training are both related to and independent of its effect on muscle mass. Lean body mass (which is body weight excluding fat content) is related to basal metabolism, meaning that the higher the muscle mass, the more energy your body burns per pound, making it easier to maintain net energy balance. Avoiding excesses in net energy means avoiding excess weight gain. In fact, resistance training is more likely to decrease waist circumference (abdominal fat) than aerobic training.[231] This is important, because abdominal fat also causes fat to envelop the organs in the abdomen, leading to increased risks of high blood pressure, high cholesterol, and diabetes. Resistance training appears to be more effective in targeting this abdominal fat. Just two days of resistance exercise a week (for 16 weeks) has been found to increase the effectiveness of how the body uses insulin by over 46%, decreasing blood sugar levels.[232] Studies also show that resistance training may significantly decrease blood pressure.[233]

Also of major importance are the benefits of strength training for bone health. Resistance training is highly beneficial for the preservation of bone density. Just two to three days of resistance exercise per week (for one year) can maintain or even increase bone density in the lower back and hip in post-menopausal women.[234] This is important as over 300,000 Americans 65 years and older are hospitalized yearly for hip fractures, with a vast majority (75%) being women.[235] Resistance exercise is a simple, cost-effective means of strengthening bones, potentially lessening the burden of hip fractures and the dependency that often occurs.

Balance and Flexibility

Other less promoted aspects of fitness to discuss include balance and flexibility. Balance, like strength, is an essential part of daily life that is taken for granted until age exposes its importance. With age, balance becomes impaired, and falls become much more common. Of the above 300,000 hip fractures per year, falls cause 95%.[235] Falls are a major concern in the elderly. Every year, emergency rooms treat 3 million older American for injuries because of falls, and over 800,000 are hospitalized.[236] Falls are also the leading cause of traumatic head injuries in the elderly,[236] and a major risk for brain bleeds, especially when patients take blood thinners for other health conditions. In the US, the death rate from falls increased by 30% from 2007 to 2016.[236] Based on projections, by the year 2030, there will be over 60,000 deaths per year in the US from falls.[236] Balance training is an important intervention to mitigate fall risks and has been found to decrease falls rates by up to 34%.[237]

Flexibility is the last pillar of fitness to discuss. Though not as important as the preceding three for overall health outcomes, it may still have a significant role in the betterment of our daily lives and productivity. According to Unum, a leading provider of disability benefits, the second and third leading causes of long-term disability claims include back disorders (back pain) and injuries.[238] Stretching and flexibility training may lead to improvements in both. The human back (vertebral column) is not straight, but made of a series of four curves that provide support through gravity and balanced load bearing. Genetics, age, weight gain, lifestyle, and lack of fitness can cause changes in these normal curves, leading to changes in load bearing, which can cause abnormalities and back pain.[239] For example, tight hamstrings might pull down on a person's pelvis and cause rounding of the lower back, changing the intended normal curvature. In adolescents, tight quadriceps and hamstrings were independent risk factors associated with the development of low back pain.[240] In standing industrial workers, hamstring stretching has been found to improve back pain and work ability.[241] Flexibility may also play a role in injury reduction; the rationale lies in the thought that certain activities require that muscles and tendons be able to stretch, store and release energy.[242] Stretching programs may make a tendon more able to do this. One study showed that pre-shift stretching protocols, in a beverage and tin mill company in the northeast US, led to a significant reduction in work place injuries, where the odds of experiencing a work-related injury was eight times higher in non-stretchers compared to those in the stretching program.[243]

A Fitness Goal for Health

Overall, trying to improve one's fitness clearly and substantially has a broad and diverse list of health benefits. A person does not need to be a high-performing athlete to take advantage of these benefits. Minor efforts to improve our exercise habits can lead to considerable differences in outcomes. People who are physically active for just over 20 minutes a day (150 minutes a week) have a 33% lower risk of death compared to people who are not physically active.[206] From another perspective, being physically active to the point of burning just 1,000 calories per week results in a 20 to 30% lower risk of death.[244] To put this into context, a 160-pound person can burn about 1,000 calories by quickly walking just 20 minutes a day, 5 days a week, at a pace of 5 miles per hour.[245] That is a *lot* of extra benefit for not much extra work.

The previous sections talked about the many benefits of exercise and physical activity. These terms were deliberately used interchangeably. The word "exercise" may conjure up images of a gym, but exercise certainly does not require a gym.

Exercise only requires purposeful movement and motion of our bodies, hence, physical activity.

So how much should you "exercise", and what type of "physical activity" should you be doing? Major health guidelines recommend moderately intense aerobic activity for 150 minutes per week along with two days per week of muscle strengthening activity.[246,247] That is an acceptable target to strive for. I provide examples of aerobic and muscle strengthening activities in Table 2.[248,249,247]

For someone who doesn't exercise at all but wants to start, I would urge you to start slowly and build up over time to that 150-minute goal. For an extra benefit, surpass the time that is recommended or increase the intensity of the activity. One minute of high-intensity activity is said to be about the same as two minutes of moderate-intensity activity.[246] That is the same health benefit for half the time; so, people who are busy and have significant time constraints can spend less time and still get the health benefits with short, intense workouts. I personally would add balance and stretching for a few minutes every day. Yoga can target balance, stretching, and strength. Certain forms of yoga can achieve moderate- to high-intensity levels that fulfil the weekly time goals.[250] There's a 'trick' to gauge if the activity you are doing is moderate or high intensity called the talk test. If you can talk, but not sing (because you are winded), the activity is probably moderate-intensity exercise; but, if you can only say a few words before pausing for breath, the activity is probably a high-intensity exercise.[251]

Endurance		Strength	Balance	Flexibility
Intensity				
Moderate	High			
Brisk Walking	Running	Lifting weights	Stand on 1 foot	Yoga
Climbing stairs	Strenuous Hiking	Resistance bands	Walking on a line	Many types of stretches
Gardening	Heavy Yardwork	Heavy gardening	Tip-toe walking	
Doubles Tennis	Singles tennis	Power Yoga	Yoga	
Slow Biking	Fast Biking	Push ups	Tai Chi	
House Cleaning	Swimming Laps	Sit-ups		
Dancing	Jumping rope	Pull-ups		
	Kayaking			

Table 2: The four pillars of fitness, with activity examples and intensity levels

I am not a personal trainer; therefore, this chapter will not include a daily exercise routine. There are innumerable websites, apps, You Tube videos, and other resources that will meet your needs, from beginner to advanced, young to old, and healthy to physically impaired. As of 2015, over 15,000 apps were available on iTunes and Google Play for weight loss, physical activity and exercise, smoking cessation, medication management, and management of diabetes, blood pressure, and cholesterol levels.[252] Anything and everything you need to achieve your physical fitness goals to become healthier is at your fingertips. Find what you enjoy and put in a little effort, because it can lead to a lot of benefits to health, physically, mentally, and emotionally.

QUICK HITS

- Find a physical activity you enjoy, anything that gets your body moving.
- Start slow and build over time.
- Strive for 150 minutes of weekly (moderately intense) exercise.
- Use the talk test to gauge your intensity.
- The health benefits are greater with more time or higher intensity.
- Strive for two days a week of muscle-building exercise and spend some time stretching and working on your balance.

6. IMPROVE YOUR EATING HABITS

"The food you eat can be either the safest and most powerful form of medicine or the slowest form of poison."
- Ann Wigmore

From Burning Calories to Eating Food

In the spectrum of energy balance, the opposite of burning calories is the consumption of calories. Eating is obviously primal, instinctual, and necessary to secure nutrients and energy for life. All species, from mammals to plants, insects to single-celled organisms, require energy and nutrients in one form or another. As for humans, we are omnivores, getting our needs by eating almost anything and everything; we have reportedly consumed some 80,000 edible species since our days as hunters and gatherers.[253] And so we might think that knowing how and what to eat shouldn't be difficult, but this is not the case. Food and nutrition have become whirlpools of health claims, research, trending fads, big money, big business, and government regulation. This concoction of groups with different interests has led to many changes in what we place on our plates.

Changes in 'Healthy Diets'

The health aspects of food have been at the forefront of dietary change for some time; however, what constitutes 'eating healthy' can be a dizzying cycle of evolving opinions. We can look at two examples: popular fads and official dietary recommendations. Some popular fad diet trends have included the grapefruit and the cookie diets in the 1970s, the Beverly Hills, Jenny Craig, and liquid diets in the 1980s, the low-fat diet in the 1990s, the Atkins, South Beach, and Master Cleanse (detox) diets in the 2000s, and the juicing, gluten-free (when not based on actual gluten intolerance or allergies), and intermittent fasting diets in the 2010s.[254] This is not an exhaustive list by any means.

I do not intend for this discussion to describe the science behind these diets, the risks, and the benefits, nor to endorse one, nor to explore whether the weight loss is sustainable. It is meant to emphasize that food trends come and go. What is popular and advertised as 'healthy' now may change several years down the line. So, I urge caution with any specific 'diet.'

And it is not only popular culture that ebbs and flows regarding food; official dietary recommendations have also changed over time. Early in the 20th century, government guidance emphasized safe food storage in order to prevent foodborne illnesses.[255] In the 1930s, publications appeared which centered on essential vitamins and minerals, and their role in health.[255] In the 1940s, dietary guidance supported wartime conservation efforts and promoted canning of foods to supplement food resources, especially if rationing was taking place.[255] Additionally, the Basic Seven food groups were published, which included:

1) green and yellow vegetables
2) oranges, tomatoes, and grapefruit
3) potatoes and other vegetables and fruit

4) milk and milk products

5) meat, poultry, fish, or eggs

6) bread, flour, and cereals

7) butter and fortified margarine

These groups were merged in the 1950s to four primary food groups (milk, meat, vegetable/fruit, and bread/cereal) and serving recommendations were added.[255]

As reports of post-war increases in chronic conditions linked to the American diet emerged, the Senate Select Committee on Nutrition and Human Needs held hearings on the problem, and what emerged was a 1977 document called *Dietary Goals for the United States*.[253] This document linked excess fat, sugar, and salt to heart disease, leading to the following recommendations:

- increase carbohydrates
- decrease dietary fat
- decrease cholesterol
- decrease sugar,
- decrease salt[255]

The report also gave specific percentages and dosing recommendations, in milligrams and grams, an approach which, in my opinion, is difficult to comply with.

Since then, the cornerstone of the federal nutrition policy has been the publication of the *Dietary Guidelines for Americans*, published every five years since 1980.[256] Changes have come with each iteration. In 1990, there was more emphasis on vegetables, fruits, and grains. In 1995, they also introduced physical activity and the Food Pyramid, which comprised six food groups. In 2005, the D.A.S.H. diet (Dietary Approaches to Stop Hypertension) was introduced. In 2010, they *emphasized* the concept of energy balance to maintain a healthy weight. From

2015 through 2020, "whole diet" patterns were included to better fit personal cultural preferences.

The documents themselves also grew with each updated version. In 1980, the report was 11 pages, growing to a whopping 164 pages in the 2020 to 2025 update. Though changes have been made over 30 years, the underlying message remains similar: eat a variety of foods; maintain weight; avoid excess sugar, fat, and sodium; choose whole grains (rather than processed flour and foods); drink in moderation; and eat plenty of fruits and vegetables.

Unhealthy Food Habits

Despite all the trends and dietary guidance, many adults in the US would still be considered unhealthy eaters. For example, the average adult intake of fruits, vegetables, dairy and whole grains falls well below recommendations, while roughly 60% of adults eat excessive sugar, 70% eat excessive fat, and nearly all men and about 80% of women eat excessive sodium.[257] If our eating habits were graded, young adults would get an F (56 out of 100) and older adults would get a D (63 out of 100).[257] As stated in the prior chapter, overall calorie intake has increased and portion sizes in restaurants have doubled or tripled over the last 20 years alone.

To me, this helps explain why—despite the breakneck speed of medical advances in the latter half of the twentieth and into the twenty-first century in areas of early diagnoses, preventive care, pharmacology, medication development, lifesaving interventions for strokes and heart attacks, and advances in cancer care; and despite declines in the toxic habit of cigarette smoking—chronic medical conditions haven't had as robust a decline as would be expected. The percentage of adults with high blood pressure in the 1960s was 30% and stayed relatively unchanged at 29% in 2002,[258] with increasing trends in the mid-2010s.[259] Rates of obesity, as previously discussed, have soared, as have rates of diabetes. The percentage of US adults diagnosed with diabetes in 1958 was 0.93%, growing to 7.4% by 2015,[260] a nearly 800% increase. Age-adjusted cancer death rates were 30% higher in the year 2018 compared to the year 1900.[261] While the death rates in 2018 from infectious diseases like influenza and pneumonia were down 95% from what they were in 1900 (because of the effectiveness of our medical advances), death rates from heart disease were only down 38%.[261]

To me, this data shows the mitigating effects of our own dietary and activity habits on the potential benefits of medical advancements. If you recall, poor diet and physical inactivity was the leading "actual cause" of death in the US in the year 2010, killing an estimated 400,000 Americans.[19] Our high-calorie and low-nutrient diets are associated with many of our chronic diseases and cancer.[253,262] So what is the practical solution?

An Approach to Eating Healthy

Just as the previous section did not promote a specific exercise plan, I'm not proposing a new diet trend nor a detailed guide on calorie counts, single vitamins, supplements or micronutrients for their supposed therapeutic benefits in health conditions. This section will not focus on medical nutrition therapy and will not detail how specific foods may benefit specific health conditions. No. Instead, the goal here is a practical, moderate approach to changing one's perception of what makes up a 'healthy' meal.

As you will read, I emphasize the term **moderate**. I don't believe in being extreme and only looking at meals for their nutritional purposes. A meal is something to enjoy for taste and also has a social purpose. Periodically eating outside the box of 'health' is okay, too, as long as the foundation of one's dietary habits is strong. (For example, does it make sense never again to eat a piece of cake on your birthday?) What we need is a strong dietary foundation. *New York Times* best-selling author Michael Pollan wonderfully simplified this concept in seven words: "Eat food, not too much, mostly plants." Let's expand and explain how a simple seven-word phrase may lead to improved health outcomes.

Eat Food: The More Natural the Better

This heading may sound rather ridiculous. Of course, we eat food, but the 'food' that lines the shelves of grocery stores now differs from that in the not-so-distant past. Food industrialization has resulted in highly processed foods, refined grains, and chemically fertilized plants for human consumption.[253] Food processing here refers to any procedure that alters food from its natural state, including freezing, drying, canning, adding sugar or additives, and more.[263] Unless it's a raw agricultural food, it's been processed.

Let us not make out the process of "processing" to be an evil character, though; it helps ensure a safe and abundant food supply[263] to feed a growing global population. The problem is that the current processing of foods for the mass market leads to loss of nutrients. Although this now-processed food is often re-fortified with vitamins and minerals, food contains other complex chemicals, and the structural interactions are not fully understood.[253] Flavonoids alone, which are found in many fruits and vegetables, include over 5,000 bioactive compounds.[264] Re-fortification to nature's standard of precision and complexity is just not humanly possible.

There are different intensities of processing, and here we will use three categories: minimal, moderate, and high. Typically, the more processed, the less healthy. Overall, highly processed foods have double the calories, triple the sugars, double the sodium content, less protein, less fiber, and fewer vitamins and minerals when compared to other food types.[265] It is not surprising that excessive consumption of such foods may contribute to poor health and obesity. In France, for example, over 100,000 patients were studied for five years, and higher consumption of highly processed foods was associated with a 13% higher risk of heart disease and 11% higher risk of stroke.[266] After more than a decade of studying nearly 20,000 people in Spain, high consumption of highly processed foods was associated with a 62% higher risk of mortality, with each additional serving increasing mortality by 18%.[267] Despite the health concerns of eating highly processed foods, we are still eating too much of it. In 2012, 61% of calories purchased in food products in the US came from highly processed foods and beverages.[263]

Substituting highly processed foods with 'real food' may have a beneficial impact. For example, a meal with the same portions of meat, grains, and plants can have a much different nutritional profile if it is highly processed versus unprocessed. A dish with frozen, breaded, ready-to-heat (RTH) chicken nuggets, with meal-kit-ready rice containing other ingredients, along with refrigerated, ready-to-heat broccoli is nutritionally different from uncooked chicken breast with no added salt or flavors and shelf-stable, whole-grain rice, along with fresh broccoli. The latter requires more work for prepping but has much better nutritional content. They are both the same groups but very different, simultaneously. Thus, the recommendation to eat real food.

How do we know what is 'real food?' Table 3[263] provides examples of foods that fall within the three different categories of processing. But let's make it easy. Per professor Maira Bes-Rastrollo of the University of Navarra, "If a product contains more than five ingredients, it is probably ultra- (highly-)

processed".[268] If your great-grandma wouldn't recognize a meal as 'real food,' or if it came out of a plastic bag or a box, then it's probably highly processed. Simply put, **try to buy food in its more natural form.** It doesn't have to be all products, for every meal, all the time; just try to change habits and to observe the type of foods that you typically stock in your fridge and pantry with.

	High	Moderate	Minimal
Fruit	Fruit Based Pie or Pastry	Sweetened Fruit (Frozen, Canned or Dried)	Fresh Fruit
Vegetable	RTH Vegetable Soups	Sweetened Vegetables (Canned or Dried)	Fresh or Frozen Vegetables (Unsweetened)
Nuts/Legumes	RTH bean-based meat-less burgers	Canned, Flavored Beans	Dried, unsweetened beans
Meat	Chicken Nuggets	Frozen, Flavored, Pre-Cooked RTH Chicken	Refrigerated, Un-cooked Chicken
Grain Product	Pre-Cooked Canned Rice Dishes	Shelf Stable Flavored Rice	Shelf-Stable Whole grain rice
Grain Product	Refined, Sweetened Cereal	Whole Grain unsweetened cereal	Oatmeal
Dairy	Ice cream, pudding	Sweetened Yogurt	Milk
Oils/Fats	Margarine, Salad Dressing	Flavored Oils, Salted Butter	Unflavored Oils, Unsalted Butter
Sweets	Artificial Sweeteners, Syrup, Candy	Flavored Sugar (Clinamen, Vanilla, and more)	Honey, Sugar
Other	Sauces	Seasoning Products	Salt, Herbs, Spices
Beverages	Soda, Energy Drink	Sweetened Fruit Juice	Unflavored, unsweetened fruit juice

Table 3: Examples of food by degree of processing

Not Too Much: No Need to Super-Size

As detailed in the prior chapter, Americans are eating too many calories, becoming obese, and developing health consequences. The average American ate almost 20% more calories in the year 2000 than in 1983. To put it a different way, on average, we ate 300 calories more a day in the year 2000 than we did in the year 1985.[269] That equates to roughly 31 pounds in extra calories in a single year.

As stated earlier, the percentage of meals eaten away from home has more than doubled, fast food consumption has risen, and food portion sizes have doubled or tripled. Even when eating at home, portion sizes have also increased. The typical dinner plate size has increased over 40%, resulting in larger portions and greater calorie consumption.

To compound the problem, the increase in calories is not from nutrient-dense, "healthy" sources. We haven't drastically increased the amount fruits and vegetables we eat. Instead, 93% of the increased calories come from sugars, fats, and mostly refined grains.[269] As a result, we have an increasing obesity epidemic.

As elaborated on in the prior chapter, obesity is indisputably unhealthy, associated with increased risk of high blood pressure, abnormal cholesterol levels, diabetes, heart disease, stroke, gallbladder disease, osteoarthritis, sleep apnea, fatty liver disease, cirrhosis, depression, mania, anxiety, and at least 17 different cancers including but not limited to: uterine, gallbladder, kidney, cervix, thyroid, leukemia, liver, colon, ovarian, and breast cancer. In 2020, we learned about another association. During the COVID-19 pandemic, aside from age, obesity was found to be *the single highest risk factor* in severe COVID infections, with over 30% of hospitalizations being attributed to obesity.[270]

As we know, excess calories lead to a positive energy balance. This positive (or excess) energy is stored as fat tissue. Excess fat tissue leads to obesity and all the risks that come with it. Controlling the number of calories consumed is the best method to prevent or reverse obesity. Even more, controlling calories may slow aging. Calorie restriction has been repeatedly shown to slow aging and to prolong lifespan in animal studies.[253,271] Importantly, calorie restriction may decrease the rate of metabolism, decreasing oxygen use and free oxygen radical formation, which are the primary agents of oxidative damage.[271] Cumulative oxidative damage to molecules like proteins, lipids, and DNA may have a major role in aging.[271] Simply put, **do not overeat**.

The prior chapter gives "tricks" to help control one's appetite. A simple way to start is to decrease portion sizes if either of the following apply to you: a) you have been gaining weight without wanting to, or b) you are overweight or obese (according to your BMI and/or your doctor). To do this, simply serve yourself a typical meal, then, just before eating, remove up to 20% of what's on your plate, focusing on sugars, fats, and refined carbohydrates. This can also apply to eating in restaurants. Ask for a takeout box the moment you receive your food and separate up to 20% from at beginning of the meal. With time, the standard food portions you serve yourself may evolve. To avoid excess hunger and to increase vitamin and mineral consumption, replace the portions you've removed with raw vegetables or fruit. This can help jumpstart the third section of these simple dietary recommendations.

Mostly Plants: More Than Just an Apple a Day

This truism is self-explanatory. Needing to commit an entire section of commentary to explain this simple recommendation might seem ridiculous to some. It should be common knowledge, right? If it is, then our actions are not reflecting our knowledge base. Traditionally, it was recommended that we have three to five servings of vegetables and two to four servings of fruits per day. Currently, it is recommended that fruits and vegetables make up half our meals.[272] It's a simplified recommendation that is easy to visualize and implement. Thus, 50% of what you eat should be plants. In the US, about 80% of the population does not meet the fruit recommendation, and almost 90% do not meet the vegetable recommendation.[272]

Eating more vegetables and fruits is directly and indirectly beneficial to health. By eating more plants, we can also decrease sugars and processed grains. The more plants you eat, by default, the fewer sugars, carbohydrates, and meat you will eat. Over 90% of Americans eat excessive amounts of processed grains.[272] Importantly, Americans consume 300% more sugar than recommended.[273]

Plants also have vitamins, minerals, antioxidants, phytochemicals, fiber, and other essential chemicals with direct health benefits. In countries where people eat a pound or more of fruits and vegetables a day, the rates of cancer is half of that in the US.[253] This doesn't imply that one has to become a vegetarian or vegan. Evidence appears to show that vegetarians have lower rates of diabetes, lower body weight, lower cholesterol levels, lower blood pressures, and clearly less heart disease compared to non-vegetarians;[274] however, there is little difference between near vegetarians and health conscious non-vegetarians.[274]

I would add one more wrinkle to this simple advice. If financially possible, try to increase the amount of organic and local plant products you consume. Industrialization of agriculture, with use of synthetic nitrogen fertilizer, is thought to alter the chemistry of the soil, and there is research showing that plants grown with industrial fertilizers are often nutritionally inferior to the same varieties grown in organic soils.[253,275] In fact, the nutritional yield of crops tracked by the US Department of Agriculture (USDA) has decreased since at least the 1950s. From 1950 to 1999, 43 crops showed reliable declines for (at least) six nutrients (protein, calcium, phosphorous, iron, riboflavin, and Vitamin C) ranging from 6% to 38%.[276] This isn't an anomaly isolated to the US. In England, since the 1950s, there has been a 10% or greater decrease in iron, zinc, calcium, and selenium across a range of food crops.[253] Reviews suggest organic crops provide higher levels of vitamin C, iron, magnesium, phosphorous, and important antioxidants and phytochemicals while also having lower pesticide residue.[277] In essence, "soils rich in organic matter produce more nutritious food."[253]

Does eating organic food translate to improved health? There is some suggestion that increased organic food intake is associated with reduced infertility, birth defects, allergies, ear infections, obesity, and more. I state this with caution, and with the caveat that this is not a definitive conclusion.[278] So summarizing and simplifying: **eat more fruits and vegetables**. Try to make them half of the volume of your meals. If you are hungry and looking for a snack, reach for an apple or an orange. Eat as many and as much dark, leafy greens or bright, colorful vegetables as you desire. Enjoy variety! Lastly, if you can, try to buy more organic and locally grown produce.

A Recap of These Dietary Recommendations

1. **Do not overeat**. Work on controlling portion sizes. There is no need to buy two burgers because there is a deal of "2 for 5 dollars." Instead, buy one for $3.50. You would save money and improve your energy balance. If you are not overweight or gaining weight, then there is no need to decrease the amount you

eat; and you can proceed with the advice in Section two. However, if you are overweight or gaining weight, this should be the starting point. Try to decrease your portion sizes by up to 20%. If by doing so you are overly hungry, add *fruits and vegetables* to meals, or in between meals, to satisfy hunger — which leads to the second point of advice.

2. Increase the portions of your meals made of plants by up to 50%. That is half your plate consisting of plants. It's okay to snack on vegetables and fruits throughout the day as well, if need be. Increasing fruits and vegetables doesn't mean one has to give up animal products if you enjoy them. Though studies show that eating meat increases the risk of heart disease, the overall risks are low, and consuming fish doesn't seem to increase this risk.[279] So, if one enjoys animal products, a practical approach would be to lessen the overall amount of red meat in favor of chicken, and even better, fish. If possible, try to buy more organic and locally grown produce. This applies to both plant and animal products. Most cattle in industrial agriculture reportedly have diets richer in seeds or industrial waste products and receive antibiotics and hormones.[253] In contrast, animals fed a diet of grass produce healthier fats and have higher levels of vitamins and antioxidants in their meat, milk, and eggs.[253,280] This even applies to wild fish, which are generally lower in calories and saturated fat, as well as lower in pollutants and contaminants, compared to farmed fish.[281] This leads to the third point of advice.

3. **Eat *real* food**. The emphasis is on "real." Try to eat food in its more natural, less processed form. Instead of sweetened, artificially colored cereal, try whole grain cereal or oatmeal. Try unprepared chicken, cooked from scratch instead of frozen, pre-fried, ready-to-microwave chicken. In place of soda, try water. The last point is an easy way to lower sugar intake, as 24% of

sugars we eat come from sweetened beverages.[272] A good start is to lessen the amount of high fructose corn syrup you eat, to limit fast food consumed, and to prioritize eating at home. Periodically, try to shop organic when buying fruits and vegetables. Select cage-free, grass-fed animal products if possible. Again, this isn't an absolute recommendation, and it doesn't have to be for all meals all the time. Moderation is key.

I fully understand that there are financial constraints, and some of these recommendations aren't possible for all households. It is interesting to note, though, that since 1960, the percent of our income we spend on food has decreased by over 40%.[253] The US is the only high-income country where spending on food accounts for less than 5% of a person's disposable income, which means that the US has the most affordable food, as a percentage of our income, in the industrialized world.[282] If we consume less, as we should, can we afford healthier options? Can we prioritize food a bit more, knowing that out-of-pocket expenses on healthcare have more than doubled since 1970, and that national expenditures on healthcare (per capita) have increased over six-fold?[283] Simply put, try to prioritize eating food in its more natural form.

Conclusion

This chapter presented easy-to-apply recommendations, with a goal of changing dietary patterns overtime via simple modifications. For more detailed dietary recommendations, breaking down food groups, health benefits, and specific quantities of sodium, cholesterol, and vitamins, please consult other readily available sources such as the *Dietary Guidelines for Americans*. For cost concerns, please search for resources that provide recommendations on healthy food options with financial constraints, such as *Healthy Eating on a Budget* by the USDA. In addition to the previous guidance, I would recommend a daily multivitamin. I won't push supplements, but if someone hasn't been able to get the recommended vitamins and minerals with what they are eating, the addition of a simple daily multivitamin can help compensate and can act like nutritional insurance.

With that said, eating "healthy" should be thought of as the teammate of exercise. Like peanut butter and jelly or salt and pepper, they belong together! Both are important. Both are essential. Starting an intense diet and exercise regimen can be exhilarating, because changes in our physique may occur quickly. In this impatient society, we may want such sudden change, but this is often difficult to maintain. Slow and steady is the name of the game. Over time, the goal is to change our perception of food and physical activity and to make a healthy lifestyle second nature and a routine part of your life.

QUICK HITS

- Fad diets come and go, and there is no need to hop on the newest trend.
- Try to eat food in its more natural form, consuming less processed foods and less fast food.
- Watch portion sizes.
- Increase the number of fruits and vegetables you eat. Plants should make up 50% of your plate.
- If possible, try to purchase organic or locally-grown produce at least periodically.
- If possible, try to purchase cage-free, grass-fed animal products and/or wild-caught fish.

SECTION II:
MAKING THE MOST OF
THE PATIENT-DOCTOR RELATIONSHIP

"Too many people I have met maintain their cars better than they maintain themselves. The human body is an inconceivably complex machine that should receive scheduled maintenance. The last thing we want is the human equivalent of a check-engine light. We should prevent, catch, and deal with small issues before they become real problems."
- Anonymous, MD

7. CHECK YOUR BLOOD PRESSURE

*"If you don't know your blood pressure,
it's like not knowing the value of your company."*
- Mehmet Oz

Introduction

The prior chapters have focused on personal choices and lifestyle changes an individual can make to improve their overall health. Though personal responsibility is paramount to one's health maintenance, it's only part of the equation. Inevitably, a person's path will cross with the healthcare system. Physicians, nurses, radiologist, phlebotomist, sitters, transporters, technicians, therapist, social workers, and other employees within a hospital setting are prepared to help a patient in any way when needed. Outside of a hospital, clinics and their staff members are there not only to heal us when sick, but to help prevent illness as well.

To be a master of your own health is to integrate positive personal choices with a physician's expertise for the goal of preventing illness before it occurs. Key milestones that involve decisions between patients and doctors are clouded in social misinformation. I focus this section on essential areas to be addressed at each patient-doctor encounter, providing information that will empower you to make decisions for yourself and perhaps even for your loved ones.

High Blood Pressure, a Silent Killer

Blood pressure management is one of the most important proactive measures one could implement to reduce death and long-term disability. Elevated blood pressure (hypertension) is commonly known as the "silent killer." Just type the words *silent killer* into any search engine and observe the return. Why has this become such an established term?

First, humans don't feel intra-arterial pressures or its changes. If sudden increases or decreases in blood pressure are felt, it is because of its effects on organs and *not* because of sensation within arteries themselves. When blood pressure is too high, one can develop headaches, dizziness, shortness of breath, chest pain, vomiting, or changes in vision.[284] This is termed hypertensive urgency or emergency. Low blood pressure can cause light-headedness, dizziness, and even fainting. We do not feel the actual pressures or blood flow within the arteries themselves; in fact, we feel anything at all. Arteries lack sensory nerve fibers within their inner most layer.[285] This is why procedures involving catheter insertion into arteries (such as angiograms) do not cause pain from within the blood vessel themselves. The insertion may hurt, since you must pierce skin and other tissues filled with pain fibers, though once within the vessel, it will not.

Thus, one can have long-term high blood pressure and be oblivious to it because you wouldn't feel a thing. As the title of this section states, *it is silent.* Yet it is also one of the most important pieces of information you can glean from regular doctor visits. Let's look at the data.

Hypertension is a major contributing factor to several serious diseases. As stated in Chapter 1, the leading cause of death in the US and around the world is heart disease, accounting for nearly 9 million deaths globally[6] and over 650 thousand deaths in the US[4] in 2019. Strokes and kidney disease are also leading causes of death. The summation of these three diseases caused 30% of all deaths in the US[4] and 29% of all deaths around the world.[6] Though the ultimate causes of death of over 16 million people in 2019 were because of these three diseases,[6] the major root cause leading to the development of these conditions is important to highlight.

Unfortunately, hypertension is also extremely common. How many people have hypertension? In 2016, 29% of US adults were hypertensive, increasing to 63% for those 60 years or older.[286] It is especially common in Black Americans, affecting 40% of Black adults.[286] Globally, a staggering 1.13 billion people have hypertension; that is one in every four men and one in every five women.[287] Given its intimate relationship with cardiovascular disease, stroke and more, hypertension itself is estimated to kill nearly 400,000 Americans per year.[288] As the term indicates, *it is a killer.*

The Effects of High Blood Pressure

Hypertension is detrimental to many organ systems in the body, and can contribute to the development strokes, brain bleeding, burst aneurysms, vascular dementia, retinopathy (damage to the retina in the eye), chronic kidney disease and kidney failure, heart attacks, heart failure, atrial fibrillation (irregular heart rhythm), arterial plaque buildup, aortic aneurysms, and more.[289] These are not weak statistical relationships. In fact, a significant proportion of these conditions directly result from hypertension. Based on attributable risk and population estimates, hypertension is the attributed cause of 30% of strokes,[290] 56% of brain bleeding in those under 55 years of age,[291] 17% of burst brain aneurysms,[292] 36% of heart attacks in women and 20% in men,[293] 26% of end-stage kidney disease leading to dialysis,[294] 22% of atrial fibrillation (which can lead to the formation and release of clots throughout the body),[295] and 59% of heart failure in women and 39% in men.[296] And the higher the blood pressure, the worse the outcomes.[297] These are serious, life-altering, and potentially life-ending diseases, which are all strongly related to hypertension.

To understand how hypertension can involve so many organ systems, one must understand what hypertension is and how it affects the body. The human body moves blood throughout our blood vessels using differences in energy levels between two points, like water flowing downhill because of gravity. In the body, this difference in energy is reflected by a difference in blood pressure; and blood naturally flows from areas of higher pressures to areas of lower pressures, from arteries to veins.[298] Energy for blood flow is continuously restored by the pump action of the heart, stored in the walls of large arteries, and then released when the heart relaxes.[298] The generated arterial pressure forces blood to move and perfuse our bodies.

We typically define normal blood pressure as 120/80 (pump/relax). Hypertension is defined as pressures greater than 140/90. There are certain modifiable factors that clearly increase risk of high blood pressure, such as an unhealthy diet, physical inactivity, obesity, sleep apnea, smoking and excess alcohol;[299] I discussed these factors in detail in the prior chapters. Non-modifiable factors can also result in hypertension in the healthiest of us. The physiologic mechanisms of hypertension involve a complex interplay between the output of our heart, the resistance of our small peripheral vessels, hormonal influences from the renin-angiotensin system, abnormalities of fluid volume regulation, nervous system involvement, dysfunction of the inner layer of arteries, and more.[300,301] Detailed descriptions of these complexities are beyond the scope of this book, and you and your doctor can work together to understand what specific mechanisms might affect your pressure readings.

The result of long-term high blood pressure is enhanced contraction of smooth muscles (within the artery walls) along with growth and thickening of the blood vessel walls, resulting in tightening and decreased space for blood flow through the small arteries.[301] In the large arteries, hypertension damages the inner layer of the vessel, which then increases its leakiness, making it easier for cholesterol deposits to accumulate.[302] There is also growth of smooth muscles with thickening of the middle layers of large arteries, which increases the distance required for the diffusion of blood oxygen. This leads to lower oxygen concentrations, which results in incomplete oxygenation, causing increased free radicals. As stated before, free radicals contribute to tissue damage and fat oxidation, which in the presence of cholesterol, leads to the formation of plaques.[301] Arterial plaques are a shared risk factor for strokes and heart attacks, as they can break and occlude a blood vessel. Thickening of the small vessels in the brain leads to strokes and vascular dementia, while in the kidney, it leads to impaired filtration of blood. The leakiness described above also occurs in the filtering tubules of the kidneys.[289] Together, these can compromise kidney regulation and lead to worsening kidney damage.[303] The heart itself develops muscle strain from the excess effort of pumping blood through thickened, less elastic blood vessels, leading to heart failure and atrial fibrillation.

As you can see, a lot happens to the body because of hypertension. There is a dose dependent relationship with overall health risks. The higher the pressure, the worse the outcomes. Fortunately, these changes in arteries take a long time to develop. Yet they can start early. Fatty streaks are the precursor to plaque, and they are present in virtually all children older than 10 years of age.[285] The fact that changes are seen young, and progression occurs long term, provides healthcare providers with a great window to catch hypertension early with the goal of halting progression and limiting complications in the future.

Monitoring Blood Pressure

If things are silent, we may not know they are present. This holds true for hypertension. In the US, 16% of adults with hypertension are unaware they have it.[304] It's even higher for young adults (31%) and those with no health insurance (30%).[304] These populations are less likely to have routine physician visits and less likely to have their pressures monitored. It's advisable to check blood pressures at each regular healthcare visit or at least once per year (if blood pressure is less than 120/80 starting at age 20).[305]

There is no downside or risk to receiving more frequent checks, in my opinion, and I, for one, would recommend it. It is not required to do so in a physician's office (aside from regular healthcare visits). In fact, measurements outside of a clinic environment may be better correlated with long-term outcomes.[306] The American Heart Association (AHA), for example, recommends an automatic, cuff-style, upper-arm monitor (not a wrist or finger monitor). Again: placement should be on the upper arm, not wrist or finger. Cuff size depends on arm size, and accurate readings require correct sizing. So, if purchasing a cuff, please look at the size descriptions.

When checking pressures, it's important to be still, sitting with your back straight and supported (for example, in a dining chair rather than a couch), and taking measurements on a bare arm (not over clothes). Don't smoke, drink caffeine, or exercise within 30 minutes of checking. Sit and rest for five minutes as well before measuring.[307]

If purchasing an automatic blood pressure cuff is not possible, an alternative can be the use of the machines at your local drugstore or grocery store. In Pittsburgh, for instance, a local news network checked 10 different blood pressure machines from major stores like Walmart, Kmart, CVS, and Rite Aid. In this small study, the "readings were very close" to physician-checked blood pressures.[308] A larger study showed that store blood pressure machines mis-classified just 16% of hypertensive individuals as normal.[309] On average, store blood pressure machines differ just 4.4 points from actual blood pressures readings, nevertheless, they are just out of range of accepted variability to meet accuracy standards.[310] Hence, these should not be the sole means of checking and monitoring blood pressure.

This doesn't imply that these self-check machines are not useful. Data actually suggests that public blood pressure monitoring devices increase self-monitoring and detection rates. In a study in England, 29% of those who self-monitored had pressures above goal and were referred to a physician.[311] These may not be the most accurate means of testing, but they may help screen a patient who cannot buy a cuff and/or doesn't regularly seek medical care.

Medication Compliance

Even the knowledge of one's diagnosis doesn't guarantee adequate control. Only 48% of adults with a known diagnosis of hypertension have their pressures at goal.[286] It's even lower at 33% for young adults aged 18 to 39.[286] The reasons for poorly controlled blood pressures are multiple, and in part, related to the inability to implement lifestyle and behavioral changes. The behavior that requires the least effort (in my opinion) is adherence to medications.

It seems simple to take a medication with breakfast or dinner. Unfortunately, this isn't always the case, for many reasons. One quarter of patients just starting blood pressure medications don't refill their initial prescription.[312] During the first year of treatment, the average patient has possession of their anti-hypertensive medication only 50% of the time.[312] What's worse, as much 25 to 50% of patients with poorly controlled hypertension, who appear to be unresponsive to treatment, are actually just not compliant with their medications.[312] It is estimated that true treatment resistant hypertension could be reduced to less than 2% if medications were strictly adhered to.[312]

If elevated blood pressure is so dangerous, why wouldn't someone take medication to help control it? One barrier is cost. Given the understandable socioeconomic limitations, physicians might need to involve social workers to help patients obtain healthcare resources. All too often though, access to medication has nothing to do with cost. One study found that seven of the top eight reasons for noncompliance have nothing to do with cost.[313] Often it involves anti-medicine sentiments such as fear of side effects, worry of dependence, and mistrust of physicians or big pharma. At other times, it's related to a lack of understanding. For example, since patients often "feel fine", they may decide to stop the medications. Additionally, if a person believes they are taking too many medications, they often arbitrarily stop taking some of them. Others may not understand how to take it.

This poor compliance with medications is something that I see too often, even in my field of stroke treatment. I, frequently, have had patients with strokes and transient ischemic attacks (pre-strokes) express hesitancy, even refusal, to take medications to prevent recurrent strokes. They often cite fear of side effects and a desire to do things "naturally" (by losing weight, eating well, and exercising). That is easier said than done. In my experience, it is more likely that weight and behaviors don't drastically change even after these conditions are discovered. If patients have concerns about medication, or if side effects are an issue, they can discuss these things with their physician and review their current medications to make adjustments.

My Approach to Monitoring Blood Pressure

I have my opinion on how to approach hypertension. For one, starting early on, I would recommend checking your blood pressure. Young adults rarely visit a physician, yet 8% of US adults ages 18 to 39 have hypertension.[286] According to *2019 US Census* figures, there were 108 million adults in the US aged 20 to 44.[314] That equates to roughly 8.6 million young adults with hypertension. We know arterial plaque build-up starts early with fatty streaks present in our early teens. We also know that hypertension is intimately involved with the development and progression of this plaque. So, doctors should monitor early and catch elevations in blood pressure as soon as they appear, prior to developing medical complications. Personally, I would do this as young as college age, by buying a blood pressure cuff or by using the machine in the pharmacy section when buying groceries, while observing the guidelines in the previous section (sitting up straight, sitting still, not drinking caffeine beforehand, and so on). If the readings are normal, great; keep checking every few months. If elevated, check again with more frequency, and if there is a pattern of elevated pressures, reach out to a physician.

If your doctor diagnoses you with hypertension, do not fear the medications used to treat it. As previously shown, this fear is all too common. If your blood pressure is only borderline elevated, or if this is the first time you've noticed the issue, and you would rather try lifestyle changes, that is reasonable. In that case, I would highly advise that you monitor your pressure, and if you don't see improvement early, talk to your physician and start a medication. Please do not delay.

I want to reinforce this point: DO NOT FEAR MEDICATIONS if they are needed and prescribed by your doctor, especially those for blood pressure, as they have so much more benefit compared to risk. If you are hesitant, try a low dose while CONTINUING lifestyle changes. Medications are not a substitute for lifestyle changes; they are additive.

The good news? It may be possible to "exercise your way off" of these medications. One study showed that after a 16-week program combining the DASH diet (which focuses on limiting calories and sodium), weight management, and exercise, only 15% of patients still needed antihypertensive medications.[315] Thus, rather than having poorly controlled hypertension, causing arterial damage for months while trying to control blood pressure by natural means, control it upfront with medications **while** also implementing lifestyle changes, with the goal of reaching pressures that will allow you to stop taking medication in the future.

The key message: checking your blood pressure and taking medications, if prescribed, are simple and easy-to-implement measures that can make a major difference in decreasing your risk of heart attacks, strokes, and much more.

QUICK HIT

- Monitor your blood pressure early and often and take prescribed medications if you have been diagnosed with hypertension.
- If you are consistent with diet, weight loss, and exercise, there is a chance you can come off the medications with a doctor's supervision.
- Don't fear medication that regulates blood pressure if they are prescribed for you.

8. GET RECOMMENDED SCREENINGS

"The best protection is early detection."
- Unknown

An Overview of Cancer

One disease that your physician will screen for is cancer. Cancers have always been a part of human history. As far back as 3,000 BC, ancient Egyptians described cases of breast tumors, which they removed by cauterization using a tool called the "fire drill".[316] Ancient Egyptian mummies have been found with growths suggestive of osteosarcoma (a bone cancer).[316] And cancer is not unique to the human species. Any dog lover knows that tumors can occur in their faithful companions. In fact, cancer is the leading cause of death in dogs and cats.[317] Cancers affect a broad range of animals from fibrosarcoma (connective tissue cancer) in birds,[318] to melanoma (skin cancer) in fish, even leukemia in invertebrate species such as clams.[319] There is even evidence of cancers affecting the vertebral bodies (spinal column) of dinosaurs, based on CT scans of fossil specimens.[319] Where there is animal life, cancer seems to occur, which makes sense once one understands what cancer is and the fundamental reasons behind it.

Cancer is, simply put, the abnormal growth of cells. In normal cells, many genes control the process of cell division. There is a balance between genes promoting and suppressing growth. There are natural checks and balances within our cells that detect damage and signal to the cell to undergo a process called apoptosis (planned cell death). And so a cell can become cancerous after mutations in promoting or suppressing genes accumulate.[320] Most cancer cells have 60 or more of these mutations.[320] For example, a mutation can enhance a promoter of cell division. This makes the cell more able to divide and multiply compared to a normal cell. Later, a cell from its lineage can develop a mutation that diminishes a suppressor gene. The mutated cell can now make even more copies of itself than a normal cell can. If the checks and balances that normally detect these mutations are damaged, the lineage of these mutated cells out divides normal cells, sustain further mutations, and continue to gain a reproductive advantage.[320]

Early on, these mutated cells remain confined within the normal boundaries of their tissue type, though they may gain the ability to break through boundaries and invade adjoining tissues.[320] In its most aggressive form, these mutated cells may enter the bloodstream and float to another location of the body where there they continue their process of dividing to invade these new tissues.[320] We term this metastasis. These mutated, cancerous cells take the place of normal cells, using resources and nutrients, eventually causing organ dysfunction and its subsequent complications.[321] Complications result from the organ that is dysfunctional: hypoxia (low oxygen) with lung involvement, increased blood toxicity with kidney and liver involvement, malnourishment with digestive system involvement, and more. Ultimately, these cancerous cells lead to death if the dysfunction is severe enough.

This explanation is a simplified example of the progressing stages of cancer. Once there is a metastasis, we classify the cancer as stage 4.[322] The higher the stage, the worse the prognosis. For example, localized breast cancer has a 99% five-year survival. Once there is metastasis, five-year survival decreases to 27%.[323] As we know, cancers are the second leading cause of death in the US, responsible for nearly 600,000 deaths annually. Cancer that is diagnosed at an early stage, before it has grown too large and spread, is more likely to be treated successfully. Thus, detecting common, potentially treatable cancers early with low-risk tools is vital to mitigating cancer deaths. This is the foundation of cancer screening guidelines.

Cancer Screening

The Centers for Disease Control (CDC), US Preventative Task Force (USPTF), and the American Cancer Society (ACS) have published cancer screening guidelines. Only a select few cancers are screened for, and they include breast cancer, colorectal cancer, cervical cancer, lung cancer, and possibly prostate cancer (see Table 4).[324,325,326] Four of which are within the top five causes of cancer-related deaths in the US.

Clearly, there are many other types of cancers; so, why do we only screen those as listed above? To be useful, screening tests should

a) be capable of finding cancer early, even before it has become symptomatic,
b) screen a cancer that is easier to treat when found early,
c) be accurate, and
d) decrease the risk of dying from the screened-for cancer.[327]

Based on these criteria, screening for other kinds of cancers (such as ovarian, pancreatic, testicular, thyroid, bladder, and more) are not recommended, as there is not sufficient evidence showing a reduction in death or a net positive in benefits versus harms.[326] So let's delve into the recommended cancer screening recommendations.

Cancer Type	Screening Test	Age to start (years)	Frequency
Breast	Mammography	40 to 50	Yearly
Cervical	Pap Smear	21	Every 3 years
	Human Papillomavirus (HPV) Testing	30	Every 3 years
Colorectal	Colonoscopy	45 to 50	Every 10 years
	Sigmoidoscopy	45 to 50	Every 5 years
	CT Colonography	45 to 50	Every 5 years
	Stool Testing	45 to 50	Yearly
Lung Cancer*	CT Scan	50	Years
Prostate	Blood Test for PSA levels	50-55	Varies on results

Table 4: General Cancer Screening Guidelines for average risk healthy adults

(*Screenings only for people with long-term smoking history)

Breast Cancer

Breast cancer is by far the most common cancer in women and the second leading cause of cancer-related deaths in woman after lung cancer. It caused the deaths of 42,465 women in the US in 2018.[12] We screen breast cancers via mammography. A mammogram is an x-ray of the breasts. The ACS recommends yearly mammograms starting at age 45, with a patient option of starting at age 40, and biannual mammograms after age 55. The USPTF also recommends yearly mammograms at age 40, more strongly so at age 50 and older. These general recommendations are not necessarily applicable to all. Some women should be screened with an MRI because of personal, family history, or genetic predisposition.[324]

The recommendations are not patient-specific. One must speak to their physicians about their specific risk factors. For example, if a woman has a family history of breast, ovarian, tubal, or peritoneal cancer, or if there is a known family history of breast cancer susceptibility 1 and 2 (BRCA 1-2) gene mutations, then besides mammograms or MRI screening, genetic testing may be reasonable as well.[325] Screening with mammography reduces breast cancer mortality. It is estimated that mortality risks can be decreased by as much as 48%.[328] Although mammography has been around for decades, there are still many women who do not undergo the recommended screenings. In 2015, only half of women age 45 to 54 had a mammogram in the past year.[329] With further public outreach, education, promotion of screening, and, of course, with improved treatment of breast cancer, hopefully we will continue to see a decline in mortality rates.

Cervical Cancer

Cervical cancer caused the death of 4,138 women in the US in 2018. It is not in the top 10 causes of cancer-related deaths in women, nor is it a top 10 cause of new cancer cases.[12] This was not always the case, however. In 1975, there were 14.8 new cases of cervical cancer for every 100,000 women in the US. In 2017, there were 6.3 new cases for every 100,000 women in the US.[330] This translates to a greater than 50% decline in the rate of newly diagnosed cervical cancer cases since 1975. The decline in deaths is even more striking. In 1975, there were 5.5 deaths from cervical cancer for every 100,000 women in the US. In 2017, there were 2.2 deaths for every 100,000 women in the US.[330] That is a decline of 60% since 1975. It's important to note that in 1975, once diagnosed with cervical cancer, five-year survival was 68.3%.[330] Today, it is 66%.[329] Thus, the decline in death rate is not necessarily because of advancements in treatment; it is largely from prevention and early diagnosis.

We screen cervical cancers via a Pap smear and HPV (human papillomavirus) testing. A Pap smear looks for precancerous cell changes on the cervix lining that may eventually become cervical cancer.[326] The ACS, CDC, and USPTF recommend a Pap smear every three years, starting at age 21. At 30, HPV testing is recommended along with a Pap smear. The exact timing may differ between people based on history and findings; thus, each person must speak to their physician for their specific situation.

Screening can prevent cancer by finding precancerous lesions. It also is essential for detecting cancer early as it is one of the more treatable cancers when found early. As stated before, the overall five-year survival of cervical cancer is 66%. When found early, five-year survival is 92%.[329] When already advanced, five-year survival is a dismal 17%.[330]

Recently, we took another step forward in prevention. Persistent HPV infection causes almost all cervical cancers.[329] In addition, HPV is responsible for 90% of anal cancers, 71% of vulvar, vaginal, or penile cancers, and 72% of oropharyngeal cancers.[331] HPV vaccines were first introduced in the mid-2000s and protect against the strains of HPV that cause 90% of cervical cancers.[329] Since the vaccine was made available, the percentage of young American women aged 14 to 24 with HPV declined between 80-90% compared to the pre-vaccine era of 2003 to 2006.[332] Still, the vaccination rates remain low in the US, at around 50% for boys and girls of recommended age.[329] Given the benefits in the prevention of cervical and other cancers, along with a high safety profile, routine vaccination against HPV is now recommended at age 11 or 12 years for females and males.[331] With a preventive strategy of vaccination against the culpable virus, and detection of precancerous lesions, along with early detection of localized cancers, we will hopefully continue to see the decline in cervical cancer diagnosis and death.

Colorectal Cancer

Colorectal cancer caused the deaths of 52,163 Americans in 2018, is the fourth most common cause of cancer, and the second most common cause of cancer-related deaths in the US.[12] Colorectal cancer almost always develops from precancerous polyps in the colon or rectum.[326] Thus, like cervical cancer, screening can find cancer early, and importantly, can find pre-cancerous growths that can be removed before they become cancer. The CDC and USPTF recommend screening for colorectal cancer starting at age 50,[326,325] while the ACS recommends it earlier at age 45.[324]

In contrast to other recommendations, there are various methods of screening. The most known (and dreaded by many because of the uncomfortable preparations for the screen) is the colonoscopy, which is recommended every ten years. Other methods include sigmoidoscopy every five years (similar to colonoscopy), CT colonography every ten years (a CT scan without insertion of a camera), and three different methods of testing the stool yearly.[333]

Now, before jumping to the decision of avoiding a colonoscopy since alternatives are available, it's important to emphasize that the colonoscopy continues to be associated with the most years of life gained and the most cancer deaths averted.[333] There are risks and benefits to each, thus one must speak to their physician, especially because choice, timing, and frequency of screening can change based on personal medical and family history. For example, if a person's parent had colorectal cancer at age 40, that person may need to be screened at 30. That is ten years before the age the immediate family member was diagnosed.[334]

No matter the choice of test, the most important thing is to get screened on time. Ideally, if a colonoscopy is abnormal, it will be only for a precancerous polyp that is removable. The overall five-year survival, if a cancer is found, is 64%. When found early, it is 90%. If advanced, it is sadly only 14%.[329] Fortunately; we have seen the death rates decrease for decades because of screening and improved treatment. There is much room for improvement, though, as many do not adhere to or are unaware of these guidelines.

Its estimated that 22 million Americans aged 50 to 75 are not screened by any method, translating to 25,000 lives that may have been saved by early detection or prevention.[335] Further education and eliminating the stigma of colonoscopies can increase the screening rate. In 2000, "Katie Couric's televised colonoscopy led to a 20% increase in screening colonoscopies across America."[335] With continued public outreach and improved treatment, hopefully we will continue to see a decline in mortality rates.

Lung Cancer

Lung cancer was responsible for the deaths of 142,080 Americans in 2018.[12] It is the most common cause of cancer-related death in the US. Until recently, there was no supported method of screening where the benefits outweighed the harms. In 2011, the National Lung Screening Trial (NLST) reported findings showing annual low-dose CT scans could reduce mortality from lung cancer compared to annual chest x-rays.[336] The population studied included only patients with a significant history of smoking. Based on the study's findings, in 2013, the USPTF included lung cancer screening in its recommendations.[336] The CDC, USPTF, and ACS now recommend yearly lung cancer screening with a low-dose CT scan for individuals at higher risk for lung cancer starting at age 50.[326,324,325] This includes current smokers (or those who have quit within the past 15 years) with a 30-pack-year history of smoking, a 'pack year' being equivalent to a pack per day for one year. They chose this population because smoking is so strongly associated with the development of lung cancer.

Cigarette smoking is by far the most important risk factor for lung cancer, with approximately 80% of lung cancer deaths in the US caused by smoking.[329] Using the 2018 mortality data, that amounts to 113,664 deaths. It's a staggering number, even when not including non-lung cancer-related deaths (such as heart attacks, strokes, and more). As for lung cancer, even with the advances in care, the overall 5-year survival is low at 19%.[329] Lung cancer is rarely found in early stages (estimated at 16% of new diagnosis), however, when found early, the five-year survival improves to 57%.[329]

These facts highlight the importance of the new screening recommendations. The goal is to increase the likelihood of finding lung cancer in the early stages, when the survival rate is better. Screening is estimated to reduce lung cancer mortality by about 20% based on the results of the NLST study.[329] The good news is that lung-cancer-related deaths have been decreasing because of the reduction of smoking. With new early detection, and advances in treatment, we will hopefully continue to see a decline in mortality rates.

Prostate Cancer

Prostate cancer is by far the most common cancer in men, and the second leading cause of cancer-related deaths in men only behind lung cancer. It caused the deaths of 31,488 men in the US in 2018.[12] The CDC does not recommend screening for prostate cancer.[326] The ACS recommends discussing the pros and cons of screening tests with your doctor starting at age 50.[324] The USPTF recommends periodic screening on an individual basis starting at age 55, after discussing benefits and harms.[325]

So why are there no uniform recommendations for screening the most common cancer in men? Prostate cancer screening is done by checking the levels of prostate specific antigen (PSA) in the blood. As stated earlier, screening tests should be accurate, and PSA levels can be elevated and fluctuate for various reasons. In the past, PSA levels lower than 4.0 ng/mL were considered normal, and levels above 4.0 were often further evaluated by a prostate biopsy.[337] Cancer can increase PSA levels, but so can prostate enlargement, urinary tract infections and prostate infections.[337] Some medications may decrease PSA. Thus, PSA levels might be inaccurate by being falsely high or low.

Screening tests should be low risk. Drawing blood to check for PSA is not risky; however, the follow-up biopsy (if PSA is elevated) can be. Biopsies of the prostate may lead to incontinence and erectile dysfunction.[338]

Screening tests should also decrease the risk of cancer-related death. At this time, data from trials do not show reductions in all-cause mortality from prostate cancer screening.[338] This likely stems from the fact that long-term survival of prostate cancer is high. The ten-year survival rate of prostate cancer for all stages combined is 98%.[329] Like all cancers, advanced stages have a lower survival of 31% over five years, though initial diagnosis at an advanced stage is rare.[329]

Given this data, PSA screening doesn't strongly fit the criteria to be included in the general screening recommendations. However, one must still speak to a physician, as their personal medical and family history may change the risk-to-benefit ratio. It is also important to consider that mortality may not be the only outcome measure. The risk of developing metastasis, for example, can be reduced by 30% with PSA screening.[338] Even if the reduction of the death rate is not significant, a reduction of metastasis and its complications is clinically important. Metastasis to the spinal cord, for instance, can cause compression, resulting in intractable pain, weakness, and urinary dysfunction. In the brain, it can cause headaches, cognitive impairment, and seizures.[339] When spread to the bones, it can cause pain, fractures, and elevated blood levels of calcium. Even if life span does not change, the quality of life might be improved substantially.

A single elevated or normal PSA level may not be of much help, though tracking your PSA over time may be a valuable metric.[340] Less invasive testing to follow up elevated PSA levels (such as an MRI) may be helpful in screening or planning for a potential biopsy, reducing the potential risks.[340,341] I favor PSA screenings, though again, I emphasize it is important to discuss this with your own physician. Fortunately, prostate cancer generally has good long-term survival, and with advances in treatment, mortality rates have been decreasing since the 1990s. Hopefully, medical advances continue to improve the prognosis in more advanced stages. This brings me to **my second key message**: be proactive and timely in your cancer screening testing.

QUICK HIT

- Talk to your physician about age-appropriate cancer screening.
- Cancers diagnosed in early stages are much more likely to be treated successfully.
- Be proactive in your discussions, timely in maintaining the schedule, and detailed about your personal and family history. This may change the timing and type of testing.

9. GET VACCINATED

*"The world before vaccines is a world
we can't afford to forget."*
- Richard Conniff

An Urgent Issue

In late 2019, an outbreak of a pneumonia of unknown etiology occurred in China's Hubei province. The first cases were reportedly linked to the Huanan Seafood Wholesale Market of Wuhan,[342] though the idea that it emerged from the Wuhan Institute of Virology has been (re)gaining traction as of May 2021.[343] Regardless of the origin, the world would soon find out that a highly contagious virus belonging to the coronavirus family caused the illness. Dubbed the "Wuhan virus," the scientific community renamed it as COVID-19, and it has quickly spread to all corners of the world. As of June 16, 2021, less than a year and a half after it first appeared in the US, the viral illness had infected over 176 million people globally, resulting in over 3.8 million deaths.[344] In the US alone, more than 33 million people had been infected, and almost 600,000 people had perished because of the virus and its complications.[345]

To control the virus, lock-downs and other measures to limit human-to-human transmissions were put into place around the world. This resulted in an estimated loss of working hours equaling 255 million full-time jobs, leading to 3.7 trillion dollars in lost labor income.[346] In the US alone, nearly 8 million Americans fell below the US poverty line between June and November 2020.[347] Globally, a staggering 124 million people fell under the global $1.90-a-day poverty line according to estimates.[348]

Throughout 2020, the devastating health and financial effects weighed on communities around the globe as the virus continued to spread. Calls for vaccine development grew louder while efforts in research and development accelerated. On March 16, 2020, Jennifer Haller became the first person outside of China to receive a study vaccine against the virus.[349] Though investigational, the Phase 1 vaccine study developed by National Institute of Allergy and Infectious Diseases (NIAID) and the biotechnology company Moderna, Inc. was launched at record speed.[350] Less than a month later, 12 biotechnology companies, with a combined market capitalization (otherwise known as stock value) exceeding 870 billion dollars, were active in research and development of COVID-19 vaccines.[351] At "warp speed", vaccines were developed and tested in mass through vigorous research protocols.

By December 2020, the FDA had authorized two COVID-19 vaccines (Pfizer BioNTech and Moderna) for emergency use, and soon after, in February 2021, a third was authorized (Johnson and Johnson).[352] Massive efforts were implemented for vaccine distribution. By June 16, 2021 over 175 million Americans had received at least 1 vaccine dose.[353]

As this manuscript was being drafted, subsequent lockdown measures went from full lock-down to nearly no lock-downs across the country. Some jobs were returning, and optimism was on the rise, all while efforts to increase the proportion of vaccinated Americans continued. As the virus evolved and variants emerged, it became more contagious, leading to recurrent waves and governmental interventions. In certain regions, lockdowns returned to a degree, and vaccination requirements for employment were implemented as a measure to force compliance. These regulations led to polarization and politicization of the vaccine itself, rather than the rules set in place by the authorities.

Since that time, a vast amount of data has shown that the vaccine was incredibly successful in reducing severe illness and deaths from COVID-19, regardless of variant type, both in the US and abroad. Despite this success, however, public opinion on the COVID-19 vaccine was and is still polarized. The roots of this debate pre-date the pandemic.

Vaccine Hesitancy

Anti-vaccination sentiments rose in the two decades leading up to the coronavirus pandemic because of the belief that they might cause more harm than good. In large part, this "anti-vaxxer" movement stemmed from the 1997 publication of a study in *The Lancet* by a former British physician which suggested that the measles, mumps, and rubella (MMR) vaccine was increasing autism in children.[354,355] The paper has since been completely discredited due to "procedural errors, undisclosed financial conflicts of interest, and ethical violations,"[355] leading to retraction of the article 12 years following its publication.[356] Britain's General Medical Council found the physician to have acted unethically, with "callous disregard" for the children in the study by performing unnecessary invasive tests. Also cited were findings of his research being "partially funded by lawyers hoping to sue vaccine manufacturers on behalf of parents of children with autism."[357] Ultimately, the study's author lost his medical license. In the years since the original article, the potential links between vaccines and autism have been studied at nauseum, and none have been found.[358]

Unfortunately, information about the retraction of the study has not permeated American culture to the same extent as the unproven correlation with autism. Prominent celebrity voices have wielded influence and misinformation, increasing distrust in vaccine safety. Social media has also played a major role in this miseducation. In different analyses, 32% of You Tube videos regarding immunizations opposed vaccines, 43% of Myspace blogs portrayed human papillomavirus (HPV) vaccines negatively, 60% of the top search results for vaccine information on social media networks (Facebook, Twitter, YouTube, and Digg) promoted anti-vaccination sentiment, and 43% of the first 100 websites found on Google after searching "vaccination" and "immunization" were anti-vaccination.[354]

Given this data, it's not surprising that a poll from December 2019 found that 10% of adults still believed that vaccines caused autism—an increase of 67% since 2015—while 46% were unsure if it was related or not.[359] The fallacy of increased autism risk has also spread globally, especially Western Europe and North America, leading to decreased overall vaccination rates. In the United Kingdom, the MMR vaccination rate dropped from 92% in 1996 to 84% in 2002, with rates as low as 61% in areas of London.[354] In the US, overall vaccination coverage remains relatively high, with greater than 90% of children receiving one or more doses of the MMR vaccine and others.[360] Unfortunately, more and more are NOT receiving any vaccines by two years of age. From 2011 to 2015, this number increased by 63% to 47,000 children.[360]

This situation was the backdrop to the pandemic. As recently as December 2019, just before the coronavirus pandemic hit the US, only 77% of parents of children younger than 18 years old felt that vaccination was important, down from 92% in 2001.[359] Currently, 11% of US adults think vaccines are more dangerous than the diseases they prevent.[359] People hold this belief because they don't see the harm these communicable diseases cause. They don't see it because the vaccination policies themselves have been so effective at reducing, and sometimes even eliminating, these diseases! Again, this anti-vaxxer movement stemmed from the belief that vaccines cause more harm than good. But one doesn't have to look far into history to see the burden of disease that vaccinations eliminated and the potential danger that anti-vaccination sentiments might incur.

Vaccines: Victims of their Own Success

At the turn of the twentieth century, infectious diseases were common in the US, as in other parts of the world, and few people had access to effective preventive measures and treatment options; this resulted in a massive toll on the population.[361] In the year 1900, one in ten babies born in the US died before their first birthday, often from infectious diseases.[362] That same year, there were also about 20,000 cases of smallpox, with about 900 deaths in the US. In 1920, there were about 470,000 cases of measles with about 7,500 deaths and over 145,000 cases of diphtheria with about 13,000 deaths.[361] Also in 1900, the three leading causes of death in the US were from contagious infections, and children under five years of age accounted for 40% of all deaths from these infections.[363] These aren't diseases only isolated to the distant past, however; we can also find examples from our more recent history, just before most modern vaccines.

The measles vaccine was licensed in the US in 1963. In the five years prior (late 1950s and early 1960s), there were approximately 500,000 cases of measles resulting in 48,000 hospitalizations, 1,000 cases of encephalitis (brain inflammation), and over 400 deaths per year.[361,364] Thirty-three of every 100,000 people with measles ended up with mental retardation or other brain or spinal damage.[365] The burden of disease caused by measles declined with the vaccine, and by the year 2000, measles was declared eliminated in the US.[364] It's important to remember, though, that this does not mean outbreaks cannot and do not occur. Measles cases have since been linked with international importations and have resulted in outbreaks (as we'll discuss later).

More recently, the Hemophilus influenza B (Hib) vaccine was licensed in1985. Prior to this vaccine, there were about 20,000 annual cases of Hib "invasive" disease. Hib was the leading cause of childhood bacterial meningitis (brain infection) and acquired mental retardation.[361] As with measles, this disease has significantly declined, and in less than a decade, the vaccine nearly eliminated the disease among children.[361]

Again, one doesn't have to look into the past to see the continued impact of these infectious diseases. Just look outside the borders of the US and take a global snapshot. The World Health Organization (WHO) estimates that in 2008, 199,000 deaths were because of Hib,[366] and in 2018, over 140,000 deaths were caused by measles.[367] Even within the US, local outbreaks of vaccine-preventable diseases still occur. In December 2014, an 11-year-old boy in Southern California with a rash was hospitalized. Soon after, in January 2015, the Department of Public Health was notified of the measles case. That same day, they received reports of four additional suspected measles cases, all of whom had visited Disney theme parks in Orange County in December. By February, they had reported 125 measles cases with a 20% hospitalization rate. Among the California cases, 45% were unvaccinated and 67% of those who were vaccine eligible were intentionally unvaccinated because of personal beliefs.[368] This vaccine refusal helped fuel the Disneyland measles outbreak.[369]

Let's not look at these outbreaks as rare occurrences. When people travel, they take microbes with them. Every year we have a national and global viral outbreak known as the seasonal flu (influenza virus). On average, the flu has resulted in 28.6 million illnesses yearly in the US since 2010, with about 447,000 hospitalizations and 37,000 deaths per year.[370,371] The flu vaccine does not guarantee you will not get the flu, though it does significantly reduce the risk. In the 2017-2018 season, the overall vaccine effectiveness was 40%.[372] This translated to the prevention of 6.2 million illnesses, 3.2 million medical visits, 91,000 hospitalizations and 5,700 deaths.[373] In children, approximately 80% of flu-related deaths have occurred in children who were not vaccinated.[371]

More recently, vaccines have been developed to target illnesses that were so common, their dangers may be an afterthought. Chickenpox, for example, caused by the Varicella zoster virus, used to be endemic in the US, and virtually all people got it by adulthood.[374] In the early 1990s, an average of 4 million people each year got chicken pox. The illness was typically mild, with the development of 200 to 500 red bumpy lesions, itchiness, and fever.[374] I was exposed to chickenpox in a pre-school 'chickenpox party,' which was common since symptoms were more mild in children than adults, and so parents wanted their child's exposure to occur early.

What was *not* commonly known is that, like other viral illnesses, chicken pox could cause more severe symptoms such as bacterial skin infections, pneumonia, encephalitis, meningitis, transverse myelitis (spinal cord inflammation), Guillain-Barre Syndrome (acute nerve inflammation and paralysis), and other illnesses.[374] Encephalitis occurred in 1.8 out of every 10 thousand cases and could lead to seizures and coma.[374] Chicken pox led to nearly 13,000 hospitalizations and 150 deaths per year. The chickenpox vaccine became available in the US in 1995 and has since prevented over 3.5 million cases, 9,000 hospitalizations, and 100 deaths per year.[375] Even more recently, in the mid-2000s, vaccines against HPV were introduced,[329] leading to a roughly 80-90% decline in HPV infections in young American women since the pre-vaccine era,[332] the importance of which was discussed in the prior chapter on screenings.

Vaccine Basics and Safety

Clearly, vaccines provide benefit and reduce illness related to communicable disease. The previous discussion touched upon just a few of the many infectious organisms we vaccinate against that, historically, have impacted our society. The hesitancy toward vaccination lies in the perceived risk, and the poor awareness of the gravity of the diseases that they have prevented. Thus, the risk-to-benefit ratio is skewed in many people's minds, and incorrectly so. What follows are data, presented side-by-side to show how low the risks of vaccine-related side effects actually are.

First, let's review some basics. Vaccines teach your immune system how to fight off certain kinds of germs [376] by exposing the body to pieces of a weakened or a dead microbe (such as a virus).[376] Other ingredients in vaccines include preservatives (like thimerosal) and stabilizers (like gelatin). Preservatives are only present in containers of vaccine solutions, where a single vial must be withdrawn, and *not* in single-dose vials.[377] Other ingredients may be present from the production of the vaccine, such as antibiotics (neomycin), egg substrate, or germ-killing ingredients like formaldehyde.[377]

In order for a vaccine to be used in the US, it normally must undergo years of testing in labs, then in clinical trials on thousands of healthy volunteers to ensure that it is safe and that it works.[378] Once approved and licensed by the Food and Drug Association (FDA), the FDA then inspects factories and checks test batches to make sure the vaccine meets standards for quality and safety.[378] After approval and testing, multiple federal agencies continue to monitor its safety. The US has one of the most advanced systems in the world for tracking vaccine safety, with over five major monitoring and reporting systems involving the FDA, CDC, the Department of Defense, the Department of Veterans Affairs, healthcare professionals, vaccine companies, health insurance companies, research centers, vaccine safety experts, and other experts.[378]

This same process did not apply to the new COVID-19 mRNA vaccine technologies, however. Such vaccines implement a new strategy to create an immune response against a protein of our choosing. Because of the severity of the pandemic and its scope, these new vaccines were tested in major clinical trials and fast-tracked for approval via emergency use authorization. Although studied, reviewed, and monitored for efficacy and safety, these vaccines did not go through the typical means of approval in non-emergency situations.

Rumors Versus Risk

Like anything else in life, there are some risks involved in medical interventions, regardless of all the testing and monitoring performed. However, some rumors of risks from vaccinations are simply false. To understand risk, we need data, not hearsay. And the first rumor we will address is the false correlation with autism.

No Evidence of Autism Risk

There is **no** evidence that vaccines cause autism. Multiple studies involving over 1.2 million children have revealed **no** relationship between vaccination and autism.[379] Studies also showed that increasing exposure to microbe particles with multiple vaccines was also **not** related to risk of developing autism spectrum disorder.[380]

In addition, while autism rates have risen in the last decades, our vaccine immune exposure has actually decreased. There are less than 200 immunologic components in the 14 vaccines given today, whereas there were over 3,000 components in seven vaccines given in 1980.[381] Thus, while the actual number of childhood vaccines given has increased, the immunologic load received has decreased.

There was also no evidence that the "other" ingredients in vaccines, such as Thimersal, were correlated to autism.[379] Thimersal contains a different type of mercury from the type that causes mercury poisoning. And most vaccines no longer contain Thimersal.[377] There have been other questions regarding the safety of the "other ingredients." Formaldehyde is used in the production of vaccines, and a tiny amount is left over in the final product. This trace is so slight, however, that there's more formaldehyde naturally found in our bodies than there is in vaccines.[377]

Risk of Adverse Reactions

Vaccine ingredients may lead to allergic reactions in some people. This does not imply that they are actually unsafe. Although peanuts are safe, some people still have dangerous reactions to eating them. A severe allergic reaction to the latex, antibiotics, gelatin, or egg substrates in vaccines occurs in about one out of one million doses.[382] A patient with an allergic reaction (or a suspected allergy) should consult an allergist to undergo skin testing to help determine which vaccine component was responsible and to guide future dosing with different components.

In those without allergies, the most common adverse reactions to vaccines include local pain, swelling, redness at the injection site, fever, irritability, drowsiness, and rashes.[382] These are self-limiting and are not serious side effects. The more severe reactions include ADEM (leading to brain and spine inflammation), encephalitis, Guillane-Barre (GBS), and ITP (a potential bleeding abnormality).[382] Let's look at each of these conditions.

ADEM is short for acute demyelinating encephalomyelitis. It is inflammation and swelling of the brain with loss of the nerve insulation. We treat this condition aggressively with steroids as it can be dangerous. Often, the cause is unknown, though it may be triggered by infections (like the common cold) or by vaccines.

Between 2005 to 2012, there were 236 reported cases of post-vaccine ADEM, 90 of which per probably causal.[383] From 2006 to 2016, 3.1 billion doses of covered vaccines were distributed in the US;[384] which is 310 million per year. That equates to one likely causal case of ADEM for every 23.8 million doses of vaccines. For comparison, there is one case of ADEM for every 1,000 cases of measles, 10,000 cases of chickenpox, and 2,000 cases of rubella.[385] When actually studying cases versus controls, researchers did not find an association between vaccination and increased risk of ADEM.[386]

Encephalitis is a term for brain inflammation which can be from an infection, autoimmune reactions, and in rare cases, after a vaccine. From 1990 to 2010, there were reportedly 1,396 cases of encephalitis after vaccination in the US.[387] That equates to one case of encephalitis for every 4.4 million doses of vaccine. Again, for comparison, there is one case of encephalitis for every 5,500 cases of chickenpox.[374]

GBS is a disease resulting in sudden nerve damage, which can cause weakness, numbness, and paralysis. In 1976, a special swine flu vaccine for the pandemic strain of the flu increased the risk of developing GBS by one additional case for every 100,000 people.[388] Since then, studies and federal monitors estimate minimal increased risk from vaccines, with between one and two cases of GBS per one million flu vaccine doses.[388] Some studies have called this slim association into question. A case control study from 1990 to 2005 in England found no evidence of an increased risk of GBS after the seasonal flu vaccine.[389] Even if there is a slightly increased risk, it is less than that of the flu itself, since there are 17 cases of GBS for every 1 million cases of influenza.[390]

ITP is short for immune thrombocytopenic purpura. This condition causes bleeding due to low levels of blood-clotting components resulting from an abnormal autoimmune response, typically after an infection of some sort, though it is described after vaccines as well. From 1990 to 2008, there were 565 reported cases in the US after vaccinations.[391] That equates to one case of ITP for every 15.5 million doses of vaccine.[391] The MMR vaccine itself appears to involve a higher risk, with one case of ITP per 40,000 vaccinated children. Fortunately, most are mild and do not cause significant complications.[391] Even this higher complication rate associated with the MMR vaccine is still less than what occurs from exposure to the disease itself. To put this risk into context, there is one case of ITP for every 3,000 rubella cases.[382]

Finally, let's look at legal data. The National Vaccine Injury Compensation Program (VICP) allows individuals to file a petition for compensation if a serious reaction occurs because of vaccine use.[384] From 2006 to 2016, there were 5,320 petitions resulting in 3,597 compensations, so causality was probable in those cases. That equates to one person being compensated for ANY serious vaccine related reaction for every 1 million doses of vaccines distributed.[384] This is in line with the National Academies of Science, Engineering and Medicine. This group estimates that there is only a one in one million chance of a serious vaccine reaction.[392]

Summary

Vaccines have resulted in dramatic declines in vaccine-preventable diseases, which have plagued the US in the past, and a significant reduction in the impact of the seasonal flu. I cannot say that any vaccine is 100% safe for every person, though data indicates they are extremely safe, well-tested, continuously monitored, and closely tracked, with side effects mostly limited to mild and temporary effects.[392] More serious side effects are extremely rare (about a one-in-one million or 0.0001% chance of serious side effects). To put it another way, the chances of having a serious adverse reaction are about the same as being struck by lightning — twice.[393]

We forget how serious these infectious diseases could be because we have likely not experienced them. In that sense, vaccines are victims of their own success. A simple review sheds light on the risks of these diseases, the benefits, and the safety of vaccines. COVID-19 was a terrible reminder of the potential impact contagious diseases can still have in the US and worldwide. In 2020, COVID-19 was the third leading cause of death in the US, behind only heart disease and cancer.[394] We certainly do not want to learn the importance of vaccines because once forgotten contagious diseases return.

I'll conclude by saying that this is a numbers game. As I showed, the odds of developing dangerous complications are lower with vaccines than with the diseases they prevent, and the fewer people are vaccinated, the higher the chances are those diseases you've never heard of could come back to haunt future generations. **This brings us to message number 3**: get vaccinated.

QUICK HIT

- The benefits of vaccines far outweigh the risks.
- I would recommend that you and your children receive age-appropriate vaccines, including yearly seasonal flu vaccines (especially in children and older adults)

EPILOGUE

"When health is absent, wisdom cannot reveal itself, art cannot manifest, strength cannot fight, wealth becomes useless, and intelligence cannot be applied."
- Herophilus

We've reached the end of this discussion about good healthcare. I've presented a lot of statistics, numbers, and facts mixed with my professional opinion, all to show that with just eight simple and easy-to-apply changes, you can make a major difference in your overall health. These are not revolutionary ideas, nor are they all encompassing. Clearly, there's an extensive list of other steps one can take to be healthy, but their applicability may not be realistic for most people in modern society.

We all would want to have consistent, uninterrupted sleep, for example, or to live in a location with minimal to no pollution, but that may not be possible. People often have no choice but to live near major roadways and airplane flight paths. We may not drink a consistent eight cups of water each day. Home air quality may be an issue; air vents may be dusty and without filters, and mold may be present. Some people may not get enough exposure to sunlight, while others receive too much, without adequate protection. Long work hours and high stress are a reality for many.

That said, there are too many health variables to control them all, but a shorter list is manageable. Prioritizing that list to the most impactful underlying causes of the diseases that burden us is a great way to make the most of our efforts, and that is what the eight steps are all about. To review, I organized the chapters in two sections, the first focusing on behaviors and decisions you alone can change, and the second section presenting actions requiring the guidance of medical professionals. The following summary re-prioritizes this list, with the emphasis placed on overall impact on health.

1. Do not smoke.

There is no benefit to smoking cigarettes. As we've seen, it's a toxic habit that takes the life of more Americans than any other behavior. No amount of smoking is safe.

Smoking marijuana is not healthy. Although the chemicals CBD and THC, when concentrated and purified, have some medicinal qualities, smoking marijuana creates combustion, a process which has many negative properties. If one desires to use cannabis products, non-combustible forms are preferable. I would caution anyone with a personal or family history of psychiatric disease against smoking marijuana, and would caution those who have had paranoid or delusional reactions to quit. Aside from that, for an adult with no psychiatric history, occasionally smoking low-THC-content marijuana is probably not going to have major negative health consequences.

2. Check your blood pressure.

Elevated blood pressure is a silent killer. Checking your blood pressure routinely, starting at a young age, may allow you to catch elevations before they cause health problems.

Take medication as prescribed. If your doctor diagnoses you with high blood pressure, don't fear the medications used to treat it. The benefits far outweigh the risks. Many people want to try a natural approach. I would urge the reader to take medications while implementing natural means of improving blood pressure, such as exercising, eating healthy, and losing weight. It is possible that with consistent lifestyle changes, you may be able to eventually come off the medications. But even if you can't, it's okay. Just think of it as one of the most important health supplements you can ever take.

3. Eat well.

What and how we eat has major impacts on health. Official dietary recommendations can be overly technical and difficult to follow, while diet fads come and go. This book does not present an in-depth nutrition plan, so I will re-emphasize a simple approach. Decrease overall portion sizes, eat more plants and vegetables (making these up to half of what you eat), and try to buy food in its more natural, less processed forms, including buying organic products as possible.

4. Increase physical activity.

As a society, we have become too sedentary. It is important to increase movement in our daily lives, by walking more, taking the stairs more often, and purposefully getting off the couch. Set some time aside for deliberate exercise: 20 to 30 minutes a day or 150 minutes per week of cardiovascular exercise is recommended. Find an activity you like, and gradually work your way up to these goals. Surpass these times for even more benefit. If a busy life makes time limited, exercise more intensely for shorter periods of time, which may have similar health benefits.

5. Pursue a healthy weight.

Obesity has very real, severe, and lifelong health risks. I would urge anyone who is obese to take proactive steps to achieve a healthy weight—not to align with anyone's perception of beauty, but solely for improving long-term health. If someone's weight places them in the "obese" category, at least try to lower to the "overweight" category. Ideally, the goal is to achieve a healthy weight. For some, this is difficult. It will take more than a quick fix, requiring small, consistent efforts and overall lifestyle changes. It can be accomplished, though, simply by decreasing the energy consumed and increasing the energy burned.

6. Drink only in moderation.

Excess alcohol consumption is terrible for the body, but in low amounts, there might be some benefit. This is not an endorsement to drink daily. However, if someone enjoys a beer or wine now and then, and this intake does not interfere with their daily lives, then I would not consider it a health risk (for most people). Be cognizant of what an actual serving of alcohol is (based on your drink of choice) and avoid more than one serving a day.

7. Get recommended health screenings.

Cancer is the second leading cause of death in the US. It exists today and has throughout human history. Late stage cancers are more dangerous than early stage cancers. If found early, treatment can prolong life and potentially be curative, and recommended cancer screenings allow for early detection of some of the most impactful cancers. Importantly, screening allows for detection of other abnormalities before they become cancerous. Talk to your physician about what screening tests are best.

8. Get vaccinated.

The burden that infectious organisms place on humans is not only a thing of the past. Around the world, vaccine-preventable diseases are still a major cause of disease and death. In the US, our culture has forgotten this truth, in large part because of the success of vaccines themselves. (The recent pandemic was a stark reminder.) Vaccines are extremely safe, however, and there is no evidence that they cause autism. The chances of having a major side effect because of a vaccine are like the chances of being hit by lightning — twice. In contrast, the risks of infectious organisms like the flu (or COVID-19) are very real, can be severe, and may even be fatal. I would highly recommend that children and adults receive age-appropriate vaccines and yearly seasonal flu vaccines.

As we've read, these are not complicated steps. They just take a little motivation and willpower to begin, but with time, an overall healthy lifestyle will become second nature.

We only have one body. Let's take care of it without over-complicating our lives. We wash our cars, check the tire pressures, change the oil, and do routine maintenance checks to keep them running well. Should we do at least as much for our bodies?

The Greatest Machine

Let's think of ourselves as a machine with complexity beyond our imaginations. Modern day space shuttles are some of the most complex machines ever built by man, with over 2.5 million parts, 1,060 plumbing valves and connections, more than 1,440 circuit breakers, and 27,000 insulating tiles and thermal blankets.[395] This pales compared to the human body, with its estimated 37.2 trillion cells[396] packaged into 78 different organs,[397] all working together to create 12 organ systems that provide life-sustaining equilibrium. Add to this the estimated 38 trillion bacteria living within the human body,[398] and it is not an exaggeration at all to say that the body is an ecosystem in and of itself. Whether you believe we came to be through evolution or not, evolving by the hands of an all-powerful designer, or through genetic mutations providing survival advantages, the outcome is the same: the human body is complex, beautiful, and a temple worth taking care of.

This does not mean you cannot enjoy life. The exact opposite is true. One takes care of themselves in order to enjoy life more and for longer periods of time. Taking care of oneself can be the difference between walking your daughter down the aisle or not, singing a lullaby to your newborn grandchild or not, seeing your grandchild graduate or not; these are life events that bring happiness and joy, for you and your loved ones. How many daughters have lost their fathers before their wedding day? I can speak from a different personal experience.

My Grandmother's Story

I am the first doctor in my family, and of course my grandma wanted to see me graduate from medical school. She was active, slim, ate well, and had no chronic medical conditions, but in her culture, smoking was common. And so, she smoked all her adult life, from the age of 14 until she had a mini-stroke at 86. She fully recovered from the scare and used her experience as a wake up call to stop smoking. She quit cold turkey and never smoked again.

Despite quitting, and unbeknownst to her, smoking already did major damage to her lungs, and what started as a pain in her arm at age 90, turned out to be metastatic lung cancer. On my match day (where all senior medical students learn where they will do their residency training), my classmates went to Las Vegas while I went to my grandma's house. There with my family, we gave her a framed picture of me in my graduation attire (which was taken to prepare for graduation). We told her I matched, meaning that I officially had a job as a doctor and was, in essence, done with medical school. She was proud, happy, and relieved. That evening, she asked to be helped to bed, fell asleep, and never awoke again.

My grandmother's goal was to see me graduate, and although she saw me achieve a milestone, she did not watch me accept my diploma. In the last six months of her of her life, her disease also took her quality of life, as she became dependent on oxygen and on narcotics for pain. Just one change in her lifestyle would have meant a major improvement in her health. Not smoking would have added quality of years to her life, allowing her to share in moments that brought her happiness.

This brings me to my core message: longevity and quality can allow one to enjoy life and all the beautiful things it brings. Through several easy steps, you can increase your chances of a longer, healthier life. Things happen, and nothing in life is guaranteed, but you can control your thoughts and actions and make a real difference in yourself. Improving health is simple, one just has to take the first steps.

I hope this approach to health has been educational, eye-opening, and inspiring. Thank you for reading. I wish you all the health in the world.

Lucas Ramirez

REFERENCES

1. Introduction to Genomics.
   https://www.genome.gov/About-
   Genomics/Introduction-to-Genomics. Accessed February
   8, 2021.
2. Saver JL. Time is brain - Quantified. *Stroke*. 2006;37(1):263-
   266. doi:10.1161/01.STR.0000196957.55928.ab
3. Kubik CS, Adams RD. Occlusion of the basilar artery-a
   clinical and pathological study. *Brain*. 1946;69(2):73-121.
   doi:10.1093/brain/69.2.73
4. FastStats - Leading Causes of Death.
   https://www.cdc.gov/nchs/fastats/leading-causes-of-
   death.htm. Accessed October 10, 2021.
5. Kochanek KD, Xu J, Arias E. *Key Findings Data from the
   National Vital Statistics System How Long Can We Expect to
   Live?*; 2019.
   https://www.cdc.gov/nchs/products/index.htm.
6. The top 10 causes of death. https://www.who.int/news-
   room/fact-sheets/detail/the-top-10-causes-of-death.
   Accessed October 20, 2021.
7. Murray CJL, Mokdad AH, Ballestros K, et al. The state of
   US health, 1990-2016: Burden of diseases, injuries, and
   risk factors among US states. *JAMA - J Am Med Assoc*.
   2018;319(14):1444-1472. doi:10.1001/jama.2018.0158
8. About Unum: an Employee Benefits Leader.
   https://www.unum.com/about. Accessed March 1,
   2020.
9. *UNM.12.31.2019 Exhibit 99.1.*; 2019. www.unum.com.
   Accessed March 1, 2020.
10. Ten-year review of Unum's disability claims shows
    trends in workplace absences | Unum.
    https://www.unum.com/about/newsroom/2018/ma
    y/ten-year-review-of-unums-disability-claims-shows-

trends-in-workplace-absences. Accessed March 1, 2020.

11. What Is Cancer? - National Cancer Institute. https://www.cancer.gov/about-cancer/understanding/what-is-cancer. Accessed March 2, 2020.

12. USCS Data Visualizations - CDC. https://gis.cdc.gov/Cancer/USCS/DataViz.html. Accessed October 20, 2021.

13. Cheng S, Claggett B, Correia AW, et al. Temporal trends in the population attributable risk for cardiovascular disease: The atherosclerosis risk in communities study. *Circulation*. 2014;130(10):820-828. doi:10.1161/CIRCULATIONAHA.113.008506

14. Feigin VL, Roth GA, Naghavi M, et al. Global burden of stroke and risk factors in 188 countries, during 1990–2013: a systematic analysis for the Global Burden of Disease Study 2013. *Lancet Neurol*. 2016;15(9):913-924. doi:10.1016/S1474-4422(16)30073-4

15. What Are the Risk Factors for Lung Cancer? | CDC. https://www.cdc.gov/cancer/lung/basic_info/risk_factors.htm. Accessed March 2, 2020.

16. Smoking and COPD | Overviews of Diseases/Conditions | Tips From Former Smokers | CDC. https://www.cdc.gov/tobacco/campaign/tips/diseases/copd.html. Accessed March 2, 2020.

17. Engmann NJ, Golmakani MK, Miglioretti DL, Sprague BL, Kerlikowske K. Population-attributable risk proportion of clinical risk factors for breast cancer. *JAMA Oncol*. 2017;3(9):1228-1236. doi:10.1001/jamaoncol.2016.6326

18. Danaei G, Ding EL, Mozaffarian D, et al. The preventable causes of death in the United States:

Comparative risk assessment of dietary, lifestyle, and metabolic risk factors. *PLoS Med*. 2009;6(4). doi:10.1371/journal.pmed.1000058

19. Rhodes HG. Measuring the Risks and Causes of Premature Death: Summary of a Workshop. 2015. http://www.nap.edu/catalog.php?record_id=21656. Accessed October 20, 2021.

20. Causes of Death - Our World in Data. https://ourworldindata.org/causes-of-death. Accessed March 10, 2021.

21. Bauer UE, Briss PA, Goodman RA, Bowman BA. Prevention of chronic disease in the 21st century: Elimination of the leading preventable causes of premature death and disability in the USA. *Lancet*. 2014;384(9937):45-52. doi:10.1016/S0140-6736(14)60648-6

22. Carol Delaney. *Columbus and the Quest for Jerusalem*. New York: Free Press; 2011.

23. 1 Epidemiology of Tobacco Use: History and Current Trends | Ending the Tobacco Problem: A Blueprint for the Nation | The National Academies Press. https://www.nap.edu/read/11795/chapter/4. Accessed March 2, 2020.

24. Burden of Cigarette Use in the U.S. | Data and Statistics | Campaign Resources | Tips From Former Smokers | CDC. https://www.cdc.gov/tobacco/campaign/tips/resources/data/cigarette-smoking-in-united-states.html?s_cid=OSH_tips_GL0005&utm_source=google&utm_medium=cpc&utm_campaign=Tips+2020%3BS%3BWL%3BBR%3BIMM%3BDTC%3BCO&utm_content=Smoking+-+Facts_P&utm_term=smoking+facts&gclid=EAIaIQobChMI_uSjy73Z6QIVlyCtBh1o3A3hEAAYAiAAEgJ6qf

D_BwE&gclsrc=aw.ds. Accessed May 29, 2020.

25. Youth and Tobacco Use | CDC.
https://www.cdc.gov/tobacco/data_statistics/fact_s
heets/youth_data/tobacco_use/index.htm. Accessed
May 29, 2020.

26. Enrollment in elementary, secondary, and degree-
granting postsecondary institutions, by level and
control of institution, enrollment level, and attendance
status and sex of student: Selected years, fall 1990
through fall 2028.
https://nces.ed.gov/programs/digest/d18/tables/dt
18_105.20.asp. Accessed May 29, 2020.

27. Overall Tobacco Trends | American Lung Association.
https://www.lung.org/research/trends-in-lung-
disease/tobacco-trends-brief/overall-tobacco-trends.
Accessed May 29, 2020.

28. DrugFacts: Monitoring the Future Survey: High
School and Youth Trends | National Institute on Drug
Abuse (NIDA).
https://www.drugabuse.gov/publications/drugfacts
/monitoring-future-survey-high-school-youth-trends.
Accessed May 29, 2020.

29. National Estimates of Marijuana Use and Related
Indicators — National Survey on Drug Use and
Health, United States, 2002–2014 | MMWR.
https://www.cdc.gov/mmwr/volumes/65/ss/ss651
1a1.htm?s_cid=ss6511a1_e. Accessed May 29, 2020.

30. Yahoo News/Marist Poll | Home of the Marist Poll.
http://maristpoll.marist.edu/yahoo-newsmarist-
poll/#sthash.MWfPeE1r.dpbs. Accessed May 29, 2020.

31. Combustion. https://www.grc.nasa.gov/WWW/K-
12/airplane/combst1.html. Accessed June 1, 2020.

32. What is fire? — Science Learning Hub.
https://www.sciencelearn.org.nz/resources/747-

what-is-fire. Accessed June 1, 2020.

33. Naeher LP, Brauer M, Lipsett M, et al. Woodsmoke health effects: A review. *Inhal Toxicol.* 2007;19(1):67-106. doi:10.1080/08958370600985875

34. Exposure to Smoke from Fires. https://www.health.ny.gov/environmental/outdoors/air/smoke_from_fire.htm. Accessed June 1, 2020.

35. Smith KR. *Household Air Pollution: The Scope of the Problem The Health Impacts of Humanity's Oldest Occupation.*; 2011.

36. Tobacco-Related Mortality | CDC. https://www.cdc.gov/tobacco/data_statistics/fact_sheets/health_effects/tobacco_related_mortality/index.htm. Accessed June 3, 2020.

37. Smoking - Our World in Data. https://ourworldindata.org/smoking#all-charts-preview. Accessed June 3, 2020.

38. Department of Health U, Services H. *The Health Consequences of Smoking - 50 Years of Progress: A Report of the Surgeon General.* www.cdc.gov/tobacco. Accessed June 3, 2020.

39. Nicorette Gum | Nicotine Gum | Nicorette. https://www.nicorette.com/products/nicorette-gum.html?gclid=EAIaIQobChMIhIP0nd_m6QIVnB-tBh3gFQS0EAAYASAAEgIUYvD_BwE&gclsrc=aw.ds. Accessed June 3, 2020.

40. How Much Nicotine Is in a Cigarette, Cigar, and E-Cigarette? . https://www.healthline.com/health/how-much-nicotine-is-in-a-cigarette#nicotine-in-cigarettes. Accessed June 3, 2020.

41. How much nicotine is in JUUL? https://truthinitiative.org/research-resources/emerging-tobacco-products/how-much-

nicotine-juul. Accessed June 3, 2020.

42. Harmful Chemicals in Tobacco Products | American Cancer Society. https://www.cancer.org/cancer-causes/tobacco-and-cancer/carcinogens-found-in-tobacco-products.html. Accessed June 3, 2020.

43. Health Effects of Cigarette Smoking | CDC. https://www.cdc.gov/tobacco/data_statistics/fact_s heets/health_effects/effects_cig_smoking/index.htm. Accessed June 3, 2020.

44. Leading Causes of Death. https://www.mdch.state.mi.us/pha/osr/deaths/cau srankcnty.asp. Accessed June 3, 2020.

45. Smoking and Heart Disease and Stroke | Overviews of Diseases/Conditions | Tips From Former Smokers | CDC. https://www.cdc.gov/tobacco/campaign/tips/disea ses/heart-disease-stroke.html. Accessed June 13, 2020.

46. Secondhand Smoke (SHS) Facts | Smoking & Tobacco Use | CDC. https://www.cdc.gov/tobacco/data_statistics/fact_s heets/secondhand_smoke/general_facts/index.htm. Accessed June 13, 2020.

47. Potera C. Smoking and secondhand smoke. Study finds no level of SHS exposure free of effects. *Environ Health Perspect*. 2010;118(11):A474. doi:10.1289/ehp.118-a474a

48. Study suggests even "light" smoking can kill you - News on Heart.org. https://newsarchive.heart.org/study-suggests-even-light-smoking-can-kill-you/. Accessed June 13, 2020.

49. Luoto R, Uutela A, Puska P. Occasional smoking increases total and cardiovascular mortality among men. *Nicotine Tob Res*. 2000;2(2):133-139.

doi:10.1080/713688127

50. Thun MJ, Jemal A. How much of the decrease in cancer death rates in the United States is attributable to reductions in tobacco smoking? *Tob Control.* 2006;15(5):345-347. doi:10.1136/tc.2006.017749

51. JUUL | The Smoking Alternative, unlike any E-Cigarette or Vape. https://www.juul.com/about-juul. Accessed June 15, 2020.

52. Etter JF. E-cigarettes and the obsolescence of combustion. *Expert Rev Respir Med.* 2018;12(5):345-347. doi:10.1080/17476348.2018.1453809

53. Boas Z, Gupta P, Moheimani RS, et al. Activation of the "Splenocardiac Axis" by electronic and tobacco cigarettes in otherwise healthy young adults. *Physiol Rep.* 2017;5(17):e13393. doi:10.14814/phy2.13393

54. Ndunda PM, Muutu TM. Abstract 9: Electronic Cigarette Use is Associated With a Higher Risk of Stroke. *Stroke.* 2019;50(Suppl_1). doi:10.1161/str.50.suppl_1.9

55. Samson K. Add Seizures to the Risks Associated with E-Cigarettes/Vaping. *Neurol Today.* 2019;19(20):1. doi:10.1097/01.nt.0000604224.25533.47

56. Christiani DC. Vaping-induced acute lung injury. *N Engl J Med.* 2020;382(10):960-962. doi:10.1056/NEJMe1912032

57. Quick Facts on the Risks of E-cigarettes for Kids, Teens, and Young Adults | CDC. https://www.cdc.gov/tobacco/basic_information/e-cigarettes/Quick-Facts-on-the-Risks-of-E-cigarettes-for-Kids-Teens-and-Young-Adults.html. Accessed June 15, 2020.

58. Truth Initiative. E-cigarettes: Facts, stats and regulations. Infosecurity. https://truthinitiative.org/research-

resources/emerging-tobacco-products/e-cigarettes-facts-stats-and-regulations#:~:text=Between 2012 and 2013%2C 2.4,among adults aged 45-64. Published 2019. Accessed July 25, 2020.

59. Tang M shong, Wu XR, Lee HW, et al. Electronic-cigarette smoke induces lung adenocarcinoma and bladder urothelial hyperplasia in mice. *Proc Natl Acad Sci U S A*. 2019;116(43):21727-21731. doi:10.1073/pnas.1911321116

60. Is Vaping a Gateway Drug? | | Keck Medicine of USC. https://www.keckmedicine.org/is-vaping-a-gateway-drug/. Accessed June 15, 2020.

61. The Path to Smoking Addiction Starts at Very Young Ages / 2 Although Stopping Youth Smoking Initiation is Best, Simply Delaying It Can Produce Substantial Benefits. doi:10.3886/ICPSR36361.v1

62. Adolescents and Tobacco: Trends | HHS.gov. https://www.hhs.gov/ash/oah/adolescent-development/substance-use/drugs/tobacco/trends/index.html. Accessed June 15, 2020.

63. Caraballo RS, Shafer PR, Patel D, Davis KC, McAfee TA. Quit methods used by us adult cigarette smokers, 2014-2016. *Prev Chronic Dis*. 2017;14(4). doi:10.5888/pcd14.160600

64. Hajek P, Phillips-Waller A, Przulj D, et al. A Randomized Trial of E-Cigarettes versus Nicotine-Replacement Therapy. *N Engl J Med*. 2019;380(7):629-637. doi:10.1056/NEJMoa1808779

65. About Electronic Cigarettes (E-Cigarettes) | Smoking & Tobacco Use | CDC. https://www.cdc.gov/tobacco/basic_information/e-cigarettes/about-e-cigarettes.html. Accessed June 15, 2020.

66. Benefits of Quitting | Smoking & Tobacco Use | CDC. https://www.cdc.gov/tobacco/quit_smoking/how_to_quit/benefits/index.htm. Accessed June 27, 2020.

67. Smoking Cessation: Fast Facts | Smoking & Tobacco Use | CDC. https://www.cdc.gov/tobacco/data_statistics/fact_sheets/cessation/smoking-cessation-fast-facts/index.html. Accessed June 27, 2020.

68. Buczkowski K, Marcinowicz L, Czachowski S, Piszczek E. Motivations toward smoking cessation, reasons for relapse, and modes of quitting: Results from a qualitative study among former and current smokers. *Patient Prefer Adherence*. 2014;8:1353-1363. doi:10.2147/PPA.S67767

69. Cigarette Prices by State in 2021 | Balancing Everything. https://balancingeverything.com/cigarette-prices-by-state/. Accessed October 20, 2021.

70. Viagra Prices, Coupons & Patient Assistance Programs - Drugs.com. https://www.drugs.com/price-guide/viagra. Accessed June 27, 2020.

71. Kovac JR, Labbate C, Ramasamy R, Tang D, Lipshultz LI. Effects of cigarette smoking on erectile dysfunction. *Andrologia*. 2015;47(10):1087-1092. doi:10.1111/and.12393

72. How to Quit Smoking - HelpGuide.org. https://www.helpguide.org/articles/addictions/how-to-quit-smoking.htm. Accessed June 27, 2020.

73. Ways to Quit Smoking: Cold Turkey, Nicotine Replacement Therapy, and More. https://www.webmd.com/smoking-cessation/quit-smoking#2. Accessed June 27, 2020.

74. Manage Your Quit Day | Quit Guide | Quit Smoking | Tips From Former Smokers | CDC.

https://www.cdc.gov/tobacco/campaign/tips/quit-smoking/guide/steps-on-quit-day.html. Accessed June 27, 2020.

75. Lindson-Hawley N, Banting M, West R, Michie S, Shinkins B, Aveyard P. Gradual versus abrupt smoking cessation a randomized, controlled noninferiority trial. *Ann Intern Med.* 2016;164(9):585-592. doi:10.7326/M14-2805

76. Hartmann-Boyce J, Chepkin SC, Ye W, Bullen C, Lancaster T. Nicotine replacement therapy versus control for smoking cessation. *Cochrane Database Syst Rev.* 2018;2018(5). doi:10.1002/14651858.CD000146.pub5

77. Lindson N, Chepkin SC, Ye W, Fanshawe TR, Bullen C, Hartmann-Boyce J. Different doses, durations and modes of delivery of nicotine replacement therapy for smoking cessation. *Cochrane Database Syst Rev.* 2019;2019(4). doi:10.1002/14651858.CD013308

78. Ebbert J. Varenicline for smoking cessation: efficacy, safety, and treatment recommendations. *Patient Prefer Adherence.* 2010;4:355. doi:10.2147/ppa.s10620

79. Wilkes S. The use of bupropion SR in cigarette smoking cessation. *Int J COPD.* 2008;3(1):45-53. doi:10.2147/copd.s1121

80. FDA Removes Black Box Warning from Varenicline's Label. *NEJM J Watch.* 2016;2016. doi:10.1056/NEJM-JW.FW112367

81. Yu B, Chen X, Chen X, Yan H. Marijuana legalization and historical trends in marijuana use among US residents aged 12-25: Results from the 1979-2016 National Survey on drug use and health. *BMC Public Health.* 2020;20(1):156. doi:10.1186/s12889-020-8253-4

82. Berenson A. *Tell Your Children the Truth about Marijuana, Mental Inllness, and Violence.* New York:

Free Press; 2019.

83. Keyhani S, Steigerwald S, Ishida J, et al. Risks and benefits of marijuana use a national survey of U.S. Adults. *Ann Intern Med.* 2018;169(5):282-290. doi:10.7326/M18-0810

84. Hanba C, Hanba D. Opioid and Drug Prevalence in Top 40's Music: A 30 Year Review. doi:10.3122/jabfm.2018.05.180001

85. Seth Rogen on Smoking Pot & Making Pottery During Quarantine - YouTube. https://www.youtube.com/watch?v=MOYBlOBhQW E. Accessed July 1, 2020.

86. Two-thirds of Americans support marijuana legalization | Pew Research Center. https://www.pewresearch.org/fact-tank/2019/11/14/americans-support-marijuana-legalization/. Accessed July 1, 2020.

87. The End of Prohibition - HISTORY. https://www.history.com/news/the-night-prohibition-ended. Accessed July 1, 2020.

88. FastStats - Alcohol Use. https://www.cdc.gov/nchs/fastats/alcohol.htm. Accessed October 20, 2021.

89. National Academies of Sciences E and M, Division H and M, Practice B on PH and PH, Agenda C on the HE of MAER and R. Challenges and Barriers in Conducting Cannabis Research. January 2017. https://www.ncbi.nlm.nih.gov/books/NBK425757/. Accessed July 1, 2020.

90. Atakan Z. Cannabis, a complex plant: Different compounds and different effects on individuals. *Ther Adv Psychopharmacol.* 2012;2(6):241-254. doi:10.1177/2045125312457586

91. Juknat A, Rimmerman N, Levy R, Vogel Z, Kozela E.

Cannabidiol affects the expression of genes involved in zinc homeostasis in BV-2 microglial cells. In: *Neurochemistry International*. Vol 61. Pergamon; 2012:923-930. doi:10.1016/j.neuint.2011.12.002

92. Health Effects of Marijuana and Cannabis-Derived Products Presented in New Report | National Academies. https://www.nationalacademies.org/news/2017/01/health-effects-of-marijuana-and-cannabis-derived-products-presented-in-new-report. Accessed July 25, 2020.

93. Fife TD, Moawad H, Moschonas C, Shepard K, Hammond N. Clinical perspectives on medical marijuana (cannabis) for neurologic disorders. *Neurol Clin Pract*. 2015;5(4):344-351. doi:10.1212/CPJ.0000000000000162

94. Wong SS, Wilens TE. Medical cannabinoids in children and adolescents: A systematic review. *Pediatrics*. 2017;140(5). doi:10.1542/peds.2017-1818

95. Whiting PF, Wolff RF, Deshpande S, et al. Cannabinoids for medical use: A systematic review and meta-analysis. *JAMA - J Am Med Assoc*. 2015;313(24):2456-2473. doi:10.1001/jama.2015.6358

96. FDA Approves First Drug Comprised of an Active Ingredient Derived from Marijuana to Treat Rare, Severe Forms of Epilepsy | FDA. https://www.fda.gov/news-events/press-announcements/fda-approves-first-drug-comprised-active-ingredient-derived-marijuana-treat-rare-severe-forms. Accessed July 25, 2020.

97. Does Marijuana Help Treat Glaucoma or Other Eye Conditions? - American Academy of Ophthalmology. https://www.aao.org/eye-health/tips-prevention/medical-marijuana-glaucoma-treament.

Accessed July 25, 2020.

98. Stampanoni Bassi M, Sancesario A, Morace R, Centonze D, Iezzi E. Cannabinoids in Parkinson's Disease. *Cannabis Cannabinoid Res.* 2017;2(1):21-29. doi:10.1089/can.2017.0002

99. Yenilmez F, Fründt O, Hidding U, Buhmann C. Cannabis in Parkinson's disease: The patients' view. *J Parkinsons Dis.* 2021;11(1):309-321. doi:10.3233/JPD-202260

100. Arseneault L, Cannon M, Witton J, Murray RM. Causal association between cannabis and psychosis: Examination of the evidence. *Br J Psychiatry.* 2004;184(FEB.):110-117. doi:10.1192/bjp.184.2.110

101. Di Forti M, Quattrone D, Freeman TP, et al. The contribution of cannabis use to variation in the incidence of psychotic disorder across Europe (EU-GEI): a multicentre case-control study. *The Lancet Psychiatry.* 2019;6(5):427-436. doi:10.1016/S2215-0366(19)30048-3

102. Fontanella CA, Steelesmith DL, Brock G, Bridge JA, Campo J V., Fristad MA. Association of Cannabis Use with Self-harm and Mortality Risk among Youths with Mood Disorders. *JAMA Pediatr.* 2021;175(4):377-384. doi:10.1001/jamapediatrics.2020.5494

103. Gobbi G, Atkin T, Zytynski T, et al. Association of Cannabis Use in Adolescence and Risk of Depression, Anxiety, and Suicidality in Young Adulthood: A Systematic Review and Meta-analysis. *JAMA Psychiatry.* 2019;76(4):426-434. doi:10.1001/jamapsychiatry.2018.4500

104. How did they make penicillin? https://www.nlm.nih.gov/exhibition/fromdnatobeer/exhibition-interactive/illustrations/penicillin-alternative.html. Accessed July 25, 2020.

105. Johnson SB, Blum RW, Giedd JN. Adolescent Maturity and the Brain: The Promise and Pitfalls of Neuroscience Research in Adolescent Health Policy. *J Adolesc Heal*. 2009;45(3):216-221. doi:10.1016/j.jadohealth.2009.05.016

106. Jesus' First Miracle Timeline. https://www.biblestudy.org/maps/jesus-first-miracle-timeline.html. Accessed August 8, 2020.

107. Alcoholic Beverages Market Size and Share | Industry Analysis, 2025. https://www.alliedmarketresearch.com/alcoholic-beverages-market. Accessed August 8, 2020.

108. • U.S. - alcohol tax revenue 2025 | Statista. https://www.statista.com/statistics/248952/revenues-from-alcohol-tax-and-forecast-in-the-us/. Accessed August 8, 2020.

109. Prohibition - HISTORY. https://www.history.com/topics/roaring-twenties/prohibition. Accessed August 8, 2020.

110. Prohibition Profits Transformed the Mob - Prohibition: An Interactive History. http://prohibition.themobmuseum.org/the-history/the-rise-of-organized-crime/the-mob-during-prohibition/. Accessed August 8, 2020.

111. Valenzuala F. Alcohol and Neurotransmitter Interactions. https://pubs.niaaa.nih.gov/publications/arh21-2/144.pdf. Accessed August 10, 2020.

112. Alcohol Poisoning Deaths | VitalSigns | CDC. https://www.cdc.gov/vitalsigns/alcohol-poisoning-deaths/index.html. Accessed August 10, 2020.

113. Osna NA, Donohue TM, Kharbanda KK. Alcoholic Liver Disease: Pathogenesis and Current Management. *Alcohol Res*. 2017;38(2):147-161.

/pmc/articles/PMC5513682/?report=abstract. Accessed August 10, 2020.

114. Shield KD, Parry C, Rehm J. Chronic diseases and conditions related to alcohol use. *Alcohol Res Curr Rev.* 2013;35(2):155-171. /pmc/articles/PMC3908707/?report=abstract. Accessed August 10, 2020.

115. Injury Center C. *10 Leading Causes of Death by Age Group, United States – 2010.*

116. Hingson RW, Heeren T, Jamanka A, Howland J. Age of drinking onset and unintentional injury involvement after drinking. *J Am Med Assoc.* 2000;284(12):1527-1533. doi:10.1001/jama.284.12.1527

117. Almost One-Fourth of Suicide Victims Are Legally Intoxicated When They Die - Partnership to End Addiction | Where Families Find Answers. https://drugfree.org/drug-and-alcohol-news/almost-one-fourth-of-suicide-victims-are-legally-intoxicated-when-they-die/. Accessed August 10, 2020.

118. Alcohol-Related Crimes: Statistics and Facts - Alcohol Rehab Guide. https://www.alcoholrehabguide.org/alcohol/crimes/. Accessed August 10, 2020.

119. Naimi TS, Xuan Z, Cooper SE, et al. Alcohol Involvement in Homicide Victimization in the United States. *Alcohol Clin Exp Res.* 2016;40(12):2614-2621. doi:10.1111/acer.13230

120. AM W, IP C, RW H, PA P. Using Death Certificates to Explore Changes in Alcohol-Related Mortality in the United States, 1999 to 2017. *Alcohol Clin Exp Res.* 2020;44(1):178-187. doi:10.1111/ACER.14239

121. Report - Alcohol-Attributable Deaths, US, By Sex, Excessive Use. https://nccd.cdc.gov/DPH_ARDI/Default/Report.as

px?T=AAM&P=1A04A664-0244-42C1-91DE-
316F3AF6B447&R=B885BD06-13DF-45CD-8DD8-
AA6B178C4ECE&M=32B5FFE7-81D2-43C5-A892-
9B9B3C4246C7&F=&D=. Accessed October 20, 2021.

122. Alcohol Facts and Statistics | National Institute on
Alcohol Abuse and Alcoholism (NIAAA).
https://www.niaaa.nih.gov/publications/brochures-
and-fact-sheets/alcohol-facts-and-statistics. Accessed
August 10, 2020.

123. What Is A Standard Drink? | National Institute on
Alcohol Abuse and Alcoholism (NIAAA).
https://www.niaaa.nih.gov/what-standard-drink.
Accessed August 10, 2020.

124. Binge Drinking is a serious but preventable problem of
excessive alcohol use | CDC.
https://www.cdc.gov/alcohol/fact-sheets/binge-
drinking.htm. Accessed August 27, 2020.

125. Binge Drinking: Health Effects, Signs, and Prevention.
https://www.webmd.com/mental-
health/addiction/binge-drinking#1. Accessed August
27, 2020.

126. Di Castelnuovo A, Costanzo S, Bagnardi V, Donati
MB, Iacoviello L, De Gaetano G. Alcohol dosing and
total mortality in men and women: An updated meta-
analysis of 34 prospective studies. *Arch Intern Med.*
2006;166(22):2437-2445.
doi:10.1001/archinte.166.22.2437

127. Corrao G, Bagnardi V, Zambon A, La Vecchia C. A
meta-analysis of alcohol consumption and the risk of
15 diseases. *Prev Med (Baltim).* 2004;38(5):613-619.
doi:10.1016/j.ypmed.2003.11.027

128. Reynolds K, Lewis LB, Nolen JDL, Kinney GL, Sathya
B, He J. Alcohol Consumption and Risk of Stroke: A
Meta-analysis. *J Am Med Assoc.* 2003;289(5):579-588.

doi:10.1001/jama.289.5.579

129. Hu EA, Lazo M, Rosenberg SD, et al. Alcohol Consumption and Incident Kidney Disease: Results From the Atherosclerosis Risk in Communities Study. *J Ren Nutr*. 2020;30(1):22-30. doi:10.1053/j.jrn.2019.01.011

130. Holst C, Becker U, Jørgensen ME, Grønbæk M, Tolstrup JS. Alcohol drinking patterns and risk of diabetes: a cohort study of 70,551 men and women from the general Danish population. *Diabetologia*. 2017;60(10):1941-1950. doi:10.1007/s00125-017-4359-3

131. Light drinking may be beneficial in type 2 diabetes: Further research needed -- ScienceDaily. https://www.sciencedaily.com/releases/2019/09/19 0916185817.htm. Accessed August 27, 2020.

132. Grønbæk M. Alcohol, type of alcohol, and all-cause and coronary heart disease mortality. In: *Annals of the New York Academy of Sciences*. Vol 957. New York Academy of Sciences; 2002:16-20. doi:10.1111/j.1749-6632.2002.tb02902.x

133. Rimm EB, Klatsky A, Grobbee D, Stampfer MJ. Review of moderate alcohol consumption and reduced risk of coronary heart disease: Is the effect due to beer, wine, or spirits? *Br Med J*. 1996;312(7033):731-736. doi:10.1136/bmj.312.7033.731

134. Facts about moderate drinking | CDC. https://www.cdc.gov/alcohol/fact-sheets/moderate-drinking.htm. Accessed August 27, 2020.

135. Children's Life Expectancy Being Cut Short by Obesity - The New York Times. https://www.nytimes.com/2005/03/17/health/child rens-life-expectancy-being-cut-short-by-obesity.html. Accessed September 10, 2020.

136. Olshansky SJ, Passaro DJ, Hershow RC, et al. A

Potential Decline in Life Expectancy in the United States in the 21st Century. *N Engl J Med.* 2005;352(11):1138-1145. doi:10.1056/NEJMsr043743

137. Defining Adult Overweight and Obesity | Overweight & Obesity | CDC. https://www.cdc.gov/obesity/adult/defining.html. Accessed September 10, 2020.

138. Grosvenor M, Smolin L. *Nutrition: From Science to Life.* Orlando: Harcourt College Publishers; 2002.

139. Defining Adult Overweight and Obesity | Overweight & Obesity | CDC. https://www.cdc.gov/obesity/adult/defining.html. Accessed March 22, 2021.

140. Pathophysiological and Perioperative Features of Morbidly Obese Parturients. https://www.medscape.com/viewarticle/703502_2. Accessed March 22, 2021.

141. Hall JE, Do Carmo JM, Da Silva AA, Wang Z, Hall ME. Obesity-Induced Hypertension: Interaction of Neurohumoral and Renal Mechanisms. *Circ Res.* 2015;116(6):991-1006. doi:10.1161/CIRCRESAHA.116.305697

142. Products - Data Briefs - Number 360 - February 2020. https://www.cdc.gov/nchs/products/databriefs/db360.htm. Accessed September 10, 2020.

143. Products - Health E Stats - Prevalence of Overweight, Obesity, and Extreme Obesity Among Adults Aged 20 and Over: United States, 1960–1962 Through 2013–2014. https://www.cdc.gov/nchs/data/hestat/obesity_adult_15_16/obesity_adult_15_16.htm. Accessed September 10, 2020.

144. Fryar CD, Carroll MD, Afful J. Prevalence of Overweight, Obesity, and Severe Obesity Among

Children and Adolescents Aged 2-19 Years: United States. 2021. doi:10.1001/jama.2020.14590

145. Average American Weighs 17 Pounds More Than "Ideal." https://news.gallup.com/poll/102919/average-american-weighs-pounds-more-than-ideal.aspx. Accessed September 10, 2020.

146. Obesity and overweight. https://www.who.int/news-room/fact-sheets/detail/obesity-and-overweight. Accessed July 25, 2021.

147. By 2030, nearly half of all U.S. adults will be obese, experts predict - Los Angeles Times. https://www.latimes.com/science/story/2019-12-18/nearly-half-of-us-adults-will-be-obese-by-2030. Accessed October 7, 2020.

148. Ward ZJ, Bleich SN, Cradock AL, et al. Projected U.S. state-level prevalence of adult obesity and severe obesity. *N Engl J Med*. 2019;381(25):2440-2450. doi:10.1056/NEJMsa1909301

149. Mitchell NS, Catenacci VA, Wyatt HR, Hill JO. Obesity: Overview of an epidemic. *Psychiatr Clin North Am*. 2011;34(4):717-732. doi:10.1016/j.psc.2011.08.005

150. Why are Americans Obese? | PublicHealth.org. https://www.publichealth.org/public-awareness/obesity/. Accessed October 7, 2020.

151. The Obesity Epidemic - transcript | CDC-TV | CDC. https://www.cdc.gov/cdctv/diseaseandconditions/lifestyle/obesity-epidemic-transcript.html. Accessed October 7, 2020.

152. Fat land: how Americans became the fattest people in the world. https://www.ncbi.nlm.nih.gov/pmc/articles/PMC300778/. Accessed October 7, 2020.

153. Fast Food Makes Up 11 Percent of Calories in U.S.

Diet: CDC – WebMD.
https://www.webmd.com/diet/news/20130221/fast
-food-makes-up-11-percent-of-calories-in-us-diet-
cdc#1. Accessed October 7, 2020.

154. Portion Sizes and Obesity, News & Events, NHLBI,
NIH.
https://www.nhlbi.nih.gov/health/educational/wec
an/news-events/matte1.htm. Accessed October 7,
2020.

155. Church TS, Thomas DM, Tudor-Locke C, et al. Trends
over 5 Decades in U.S. Occupation-Related Physical
Activity and Their Associations with Obesity. Lucia A,
ed. *PLoS One*. 2011;6(5):e19657.
doi:10.1371/journal.pone.0019657

156. Adult Obesity Causes & Consequences | Overweight
& Obesity | CDC.
https://www.cdc.gov/obesity/adult/causes.html.
Accessed October 10, 2020.

157. Masters RK, Reither EN, Powers DA, Yang YC, Burger
AE, Link BG. The impact of obesity on US mortality
levels: The importance of age and cohort factors in
population estimates. *Am J Public Health*.
2013;103(10):1895-1901. doi:10.2105/AJPH.2013.301379

158. Mitchell NS, Catenacci VA, Wyatt HR, Hill JO.
Obesity: Overview of an epidemic. *Psychiatr Clin North
Am*. 2011;34(4):717-732. doi:10.1016/j.psc.2011.08.005

159. Bhupathiraju SN, Hu FB. Epidemiology of obesity and
diabetes and their cardiovascular complications. *Circ
Res*. 2016;118(11):1723-1735.
doi:10.1161/CIRCRESAHA.115.306825

160. Narayan KMV, Boyle JP, Thompson TJ, Gregg EW,
Williamson DF. Effect of BMI on lifetime risk for
diabetes in the U.S. *Diabetes Care*. 2007;30(6):1562-1566.
doi:10.2337/dc06-2544

161. Feingold KR, Grunfeld C. *Obesity and Dyslipidemia.* MDText.com, Inc.; 2000. http://www.ncbi.nlm.nih.gov/pubmed/26247088. Accessed October 10, 2020.

162. Turpie AGG, Bauer KA, Eriksson BI, Lassen MR. Overweight and obesity as determinants of cardiovascular risk: The Framingham experience. *Arch Intern Med.* 2002;162(16):1867-1872. doi:10.1001/archinte.162.16.1867

163. Bhaskaran K, Douglas I, Forbes H, Dos-Santos-Silva I, Leon DA, Smeeth L. Body-mass index and risk of 22 specific cancers: A population-based cohort study of 5. 24 million UK adults. *Lancet.* 2014;384(9945):755-765. doi:10.1016/S0140-6736(14)60892-8

164. Obesity and Cancer Fact Sheet - National Cancer Institute. https://www.cancer.gov/about-cancer/causes-prevention/risk/obesity/obesity-fact-sheet. Accessed October 23, 2020.

165. Engmann NJ, Golmakani MK, Miglioretti DL, Sprague BL, Kerlikowske K. Population-attributable risk proportion of clinical risk factors for breast cancer. *JAMA Oncol.* 2017;3(9):1228-1236. doi:10.1001/jamaoncol.2016.6326

166. Bardou M, Barkun AN, Martel M. Obesity and colorectal cancer. *Gut.* 2013;62(6):933-947. doi:10.1136/gutjnl-2013-304701

167. FastStats - Chronic Liver Disease or Cirrhosis. https://www.cdc.gov/nchs/fastats/liver-disease.htm. Accessed October 23, 2020.

168. Setiawan VW, Stram DO, Porcel J, Lu SC, Le Marchand L, Noureddin M. Prevalence of chronic liver disease and cirrhosis by underlying cause in understudied ethnic groups: The multiethnic cohort. *Hepatology.* 2016;64(6):1969-1977. doi:10.1002/hep.28677

169. Sarwar R, Pierce N, Koppe S. Obesity and nonalcoholic fatty liver disease: Current perspectives. *Diabetes, Metab Syndr Obes Targets Ther*. 2018;11:533-542. doi:10.2147/DMSO.S146339

170. Ma Y, Ajnakina O, Steptoe A, Cadar D. Higher risk of dementia in English older individuals who are overweight or obese. *Int J Epidemiol*. June 2020. doi:10.1093/ije/dyaa099

171. Veronese N, Facchini S, Stubbs B, et al. Weight loss is associated with improvements in cognitive function among overweight and obese people: A systematic review and meta-analysis. *Neurosci Biobehav Rev*. 2017;72:87-94. doi:10.1016/j.neubiorev.2016.11.017

172. Petry NM, Barry D, Pietrzak RH, Wagner JA. Overweight and obesity are associated with psychiatric disorders: Results from the national epidemiologic survey on alcohol and related conditions. *Psychosom Med*. 2008;70(3):288-297. doi:10.1097/PSY.0b013e3181651651

173. Luppino FS, De Wit LM, Bouvy PF, et al. Overweight, obesity, and depression: A systematic review and meta-analysis of longitudinal studies. *Arch Gen Psychiatry*. 2010;67(3):220-229. doi:10.1001/archgenpsychiatry.2010.2

174. Carpenter KM, Hasin DS, Allison DB, Faith MS. *A B S T R A C T Relationships Between Obesity and DSM-IV Major Depressive Disorder, Suicide Ideation, and Suicide Attempts: Results From a General Population Study*. Vol 90.; 2000.

175. Aune D, Sen A, Prasad M, et al. BMI and all cause mortality: Systematic review and non-linear dose-response meta-analysis of 230 cohort studies with 3.74 million deaths among 30.3 million participants. *BMJ*. 2016;353. doi:10.1136/bmj.i2156

176. Adele Shows Off Her 100-Lb. Weight Loss in New 'SNL' Promo Teaser | ExtraTV.com. https://extratv.com/2020/10/23/adele-shows-off-her-100-lb-weight-loss-in-new-snl-promo-teaser/. Accessed October 23, 2020.

177. Adele's Friend Says Weight Loss Discussion 'Missing the Point' | PEOPLE.com. https://people.com/music/adeles-friend-says-those-focused-on-her-weight-loss-are-missing-the-point-its-the-voice/. Accessed October 23, 2020.

178. What Jillian Michaels got wrong about Lizzo and body positivity - Vox. https://www.vox.com/culture/2020/1/15/21060692/lizzo-jillian-michaels-body-positivity-backlash. Accessed October 23, 2020.

179. People Are Not OK With These Cosmopolitan Covers That Ignore The Relationship Between Obesity And Covid | Bored Panda. https://www.boredpanda.com/plus-size-women-cosmopolitan-cover-obesity-negative-people-reactions/?utm_source=google&utm_medium=organic&utm_campaign=organic. Accessed March 14, 2021.

180. Leyden E, Hanson P, Halder L, et al. Older age does not influence the success of weight loss through the implementation of lifestyle modification. *Clin Endocrinol (Oxf)*. 2021;94(2):204-209. doi:10.1111/cen.14354

181. Starbucks Coffee on Instagram: "We noticed that college students across the country are getting creative with their favorite drinks. So we looked into it and discovered…." https://www.instagram.com/p/Bm3lucSBIuO/?taken-by=starbucks. Accessed November 7, 2020.

182. White Chocolate Mocha Frappuccino® Blended

Beverage: Starbucks Coffee Company. https://www.starbucks.com/menu/product/428/iced?parent=%2Fdrinks%2Ffrappuccino-blended-beverages%2Fcoffee-frappuccino. Accessed November 7, 2020.

183. Calories Burned Running Calculator - Calories Burned HQ. https://caloriesburnedhq.com/calories-burned-running/. Accessed November 7, 2020.

184. Wehling H, Lusher J. People with a body mass index ⬛30 under-report their dietary intake: A systematic review. *J Health Psychol*. 2019;24(14):2042-2059. doi:10.1177/1359105317714318

185. Get the Facts: Sugar-Sweetened Beverages and Consumption | Nutrition | CDC. https://www.cdc.gov/nutrition/data-statistics/sugar-sweetened-beverages-intake.html. Accessed November 7, 2020.

186. Coffee Statistics. https://www.e-importz.com/coffee-statistics.php. Accessed November 7, 2020.

187. Salad Consumption in the U.S. What we eat in America, NHANES 2011-2014. https://www.ars.usda.gov/ARSUserFiles/80400530/pdf/DBrief/19_Salad_consumption_2011_2014.pdf. Accessed November 7, 2020.

188. Davy BM, Dennis EA, Dengo AL, Wilson KL, Davy KP. Water Consumption Reduces Energy Intake at a Breakfast Meal in Obese Older Adults. *J Am Diet Assoc*. 2008;108(7):1236-1239. doi:10.1016/j.jada.2008.04.013

189. Zhu Y, Hollis JH. Increasing the number of chews before swallowing reduces meal size in normal-weight, overweight, and obese adults. *J Acad Nutr Diet*. 2014;114(6):926-931. doi:10.1016/j.jand.2013.08.020

190. Xu J, Xiao X, Li Y, et al. The effect of gum chewing on blood GLP-1 concentration in fasted, healthy, non-

obese men. *Endocrine.* 2015;50(1):93-98.
doi:10.1007/s12020-015-0566-1

191. Benton D. Portion Size: What We Know and What We
Need to Know. *Crit Rev Food Sci Nutr.* 2015;55(7):988-
1004. doi:10.1080/10408398.2012.679980

192. McClain AD, Van Den Bos W, Matheson D, Desai M,
McClure SM, Robinson TN. Visual illusions and plate
design: The effects of plate rim widths and rim
coloring on perceived food portion size. *Int J Obes.*
2014;38(5):657-662. doi:10.1038/ijo.2013.169

193. Wansink B, van Ittersum K. Portion size me: Plate-size
induced consumption norms and win-win solutions
for reducing food intake and waste. *J Exp Psychol Appl.*
2013;19(4):320-332. doi:10.1037/a0035053

194. Parr EB, Camera DM, Areta JL, et al. Alcohol ingestion
impairs maximal post-exercise rates of myofibrillar
protein synthesis following a single bout of concurrent
training. *PLoS One.* 2014;9(2).
doi:10.1371/journal.pone.0088384

195. Suter PM. *Topics in Clinical Nutrition Effects of Alcohol
on Energy Metabolism and Body Weight Regulation: Is
Alcohol a Risk Factor for Obesity?*; 1997.
https://academic.oup.com/nutritionreviews/article/
55/5/157/1813978. Accessed November 19, 2020.

196. Weight Loss Study: Keeping a Food Diary Helps Shed
Extra Pounds.
https://www.webmd.com/diet/news/20080708/kee
ping-food-diary-helps-lose-weight. Accessed
November 7, 2020.

197. Decade in review: Number of U.S. renters surpasses
100 million - HousingWire.
https://www.housingwire.com/articles/decade-in-
review-number-of-u-s-renters-surpasses-100-million/.
Accessed March 22, 2021.

198. NMHC | Quick Facts: Resident Demographics. https://www.nmhc.org/research-insight/quick-facts-figures/quick-facts-resident-demographics/. Accessed March 22, 2021.

199. Stair Climbing vs Running: Benefits of 2 Exercises in 2020. https://www.runsociety.com/training/stair-climbing-vs-running/. Accessed March 22, 2021.

200. Center for Health Statistics N. *Vital and Health Statistics Series 11, Number 252 October 2012.*; 2007.

201. Drivers spend an average of 17 hours a year searching for parking spots. https://www.usatoday.com/story/money/2017/07/12/parking-pain-causes-financial-and-personal-strain/467637001/. Accessed March 22, 2021.

202. Yang L, Cao C, Kantor ED, et al. Trends in Sedentary Behavior among the US Population, 2001-2016. *JAMA - J Am Med Assoc.* 2019;321(16):1587-1597. doi:10.1001/jama.2019.3636

203. Calories Burned Standing vs. Sitting: Chart, Benefits, Risks, Tips. https://www.healthline.com/health/fitness-exercise/calories-burned-standing#comparison-chart. Accessed March 22, 2021.

204. Tipton CM. The history of "Exercise Is Medicine" in ancient civilizations. *Adv Physiol Educ.* 2015;38(2):109-117. doi:10.1152/advan.00136.2013

205. Kraus WE, Houmard JA, Duscha BD, et al. Effects of the Amount and Intensity of Exercise on Plasma Lipoproteins. *N Engl J Med.* 2002;347(19):1483-1492. doi:10.1056/NEJMoa020194

206. HHS. *Physical Activity Guidelines for Americans 2 Nd Edition.*

207. Colberg SR, Sigal RJ, Yardley JE, et al. Physical activity/exercise and diabetes: A position statement of

the American Diabetes Association. *Diabetes Care.* 2016;39(11):2065-2079. doi:10.2337/dc16-1728

208. Nystoriak MA, Bhatnagar A. Cardiovascular Effects and Benefits of Exercise. *Front Cardiovasc Med.* 2018;5:135. doi:10.3389/fcvm.2018.00135

209. Fagard RH. Exercise characteristics and the blood pressure response to dynamic physical training. In: *Medicine and Science in Sports and Exercise.* Vol 33. American College of Sports Medicine; 2001. doi:10.1097/00005768-200106001-00018

210. Hambrecht R, Niebauer J, Marburger C, et al. Various intensities of leisure time physical activity in patients with coronary artery disease: Effects on cardiorespiratory fitness and progression of coronary atherosclerotic lesions. *J Am Coll Cardiol.* 1993;22(2):468-477. doi:10.1016/0735-1097(93)90051-2

211. Li J, Siegrist J. Physical activity and risk of cardiovascular disease-a meta-analysis of prospective cohort studies. *Int J Environ Res Public Health.* 2012;9(2):391-407. doi:10.3390/ijerph9020391

212. Physical Activity and Cancer Fact Sheet - National Cancer Institute. https://www.cancer.gov/about-cancer/causes-prevention/risk/obesity/physical-activity-fact-sheet#r2. Accessed December 3, 2020.

213. Schmid D, Ricci C, Behrens G, Leitzmann MF. Does smoking influence the physical activity and lung cancer relation? A systematic review and meta-analysis. *Eur J Epidemiol.* 2016;31(12):1173-1190. doi:10.1007/s10654-016-0186-y

214. Pizot C, Boniol M, Mullie P, et al. Physical activity, hormone replacement therapy and breast cancer risk: A meta-analysis of prospective studies. *Eur J Cancer.* 2016;52:138-154. doi:10.1016/j.ejca.2015.10.063

215. Mctiernan A, Friedenreich CM, Katzmarzyk PT, et al.

Physical Activity in Cancer Prevention and Survival: A Systematic Review. *Med Sci Sports Exerc.* 2019;51(6):1252-1261. doi:10.1249/MSS.0000000000001937

216. Blumenthal JA, Smith PJ, Mabe S, et al. Lifestyle and neurocognition in older adults with cognitive impairments: A randomized trial. *Neurology.* 2019;92(3):E212-E223. doi:10.1212/WNL.0000000000006784

217. Executive Functions | Memory and Aging Center. https://memory.ucsf.edu/symptoms/executive-functions. Accessed December 3, 2020.

218. Stern Y, Mackay-Brandt A, Lee S, et al. Effect of aerobic exercise on cognition in younger adults: A randomized clinical trial. *Neurology.* 2019;92(9):E905-E916. doi:10.1212/WNL.0000000000007003

219. Rovio S, Kåreholt I, Helkala EL, et al. Leisure-time physical activity at midlife and the risk of dementia and Alzheimer's disease. *Lancet Neurol.* 2005;4(11):705-711. doi:10.1016/S1474-4422(05)70198-8

220. Andel R, Crowe M, Pedersen NL, Fratiglioni L, Johansson B, Gatz M. Physical Exercise at Midlife and Risk of Dementia Three Decades Later: A Population-Based Study of Swedish Twins. *Journals Gerontol Ser A.* 2008;63(1):62-66. doi:10.1093/gerona/63.1.62

221. NIMH » Major Depression. https://www.nimh.nih.gov/health/statistics/major-depression.shtml. Accessed December 4, 2020.

222. Products - Data Briefs - Number 303 - February 2018. https://www.cdc.gov/nchs/products/databriefs/db303.htm. Accessed December 4, 2020.

223. Depression is increasing among U.S. teens | Pew Research Center. https://www.pewresearch.org/fact-tank/2019/07/12/a-growing-number-of-american-

teenagers-particularly-girls-are-facing-depression/.
Accessed December 4, 2020.

224. 35 minutes of exercise may protect those at risk for
depression – Harvard Gazette.
https://news.harvard.edu/gazette/story/2019/11/p
hysical-activity-may-protect-those-at-risk-for-
depression/. Accessed December 4, 2020.

225. Choi KW, Zheutlin AB, Karlson RA, et al. Physical
activity offsets genetic risk for incident depression
assessed via electronic health records in a biobank
cohort study. *Depress Anxiety*. 2020;37(2):106-114.
doi:10.1002/da.22967

226. Morres ID, Hatzigeorgiadis A, Stathi A, et al. Aerobic
exercise for adult patients with major depressive
disorder in mental health services: A systematic
review and meta-analysis. *Depress Anxiety*.
2019;36(1):39-53. doi:10.1002/da.22842

227. Netz Y. Is the Comparison between exercise and
pharmacologic treatment of depression in the clinical
practice guideline of the American college of
physicians evidence-based? *Front Pharmacol*.
2017;8(MAY). doi:10.3389/fphar.2017.00257

228. Reel JJ, Greenleaf C, Baker WK, et al. Relations of body
concerns and exercise behavior: A meta-analysis.
Psychol Rep. 2007;101(3 I):927-942.
doi:10.2466/PR0.101.3.927-942

229. Strickland JC, Smith MA. The anxiolytic effects of
resistance exercise. *Front Psychol*. 2014;5(JUL):753.
doi:10.3389/fpsyg.2014.00753

230. Fiatarone Singh MA, Gates N, Saigal N, et al. The
Study of Mental and Resistance Training (SMART)
Study-Resistance Training and/or Cognitive Training
in Mild Cognitive Impairment: A Randomized,
Double-Blind, Double-Sham Controlled Trial. *J Am*

Med Dir Assoc. 2014;15(12):873-880. doi:10.1016/j.jamda.2014.09.010

231. Mekary RA, Grøntved A, Despres JP, et al. Weight training, aerobic physical activities, and long-term waist circumference change in men. *Obesity.* 2015;23(2):461-467. doi:10.1002/oby.20949

232. Ibañez J, Izquierdo M, Argüelles I, et al. Twice-weekly progressive resistance training decreases abdominal fat and improves insulin sensitivity in older men with type 2 diabetes. *Diabetes Care.* 2005;28(3):662-667. doi:10.2337/diacare.28.3.662

233. Cornelissen VA, Fagard RH, Coeckelberghs E, Vanhees L. Impact of resistance training on blood pressure and other cardiovascular risk factors: A meta-analysis of randomized, controlled trials. *Hypertension.* 2011;58(5):950-958. doi:10.1161/HYPERTENSIONAHA.111.177071

234. Hong AR, Kim SW. Effects of resistance exercise on bone health. *Endocrinol Metab.* 2018;33(4):435-444. doi:10.3803/EnM.2018.33.4.435

235. Hip Fractures Among Older Adults | Home and Recreational Safety | CDC Injury Center. https://www.cdc.gov/homeandrecreationalsafety/falls/adulthipfx.html. Accessed January 13, 2021.

236. Important Facts about Falls | Home and Recreational Safety | CDC Injury Center. https://www.cdc.gov/homeandrecreationalsafety/falls/adultfalls.html. Accessed January 13, 2021.

237. Ng CACM, Fairhall N, Wallbank G, Tiedemann A, Michaleff ZA, Sherrington C. Exercise for falls prevention in community-dwelling older adults: Trial and participant characteristics, interventions and bias in clinical trials from a systematic review. *BMJ Open Sport Exerc Med.* 2019;5(1). doi:10.1136/bmjsem-2019-

238. Ten-year review of Unum's disability claims shows trends in workplace absences | Unum. https://www.unum.com/about/newsroom/2018/may/ten-year-review-of-unums-disability-claims-shows-trends-in-workplace-absences. Accessed January 15, 2021.

239. Low Back Pain Fact Sheet | National Institute of Neurological Disorders and Stroke. https://www.ninds.nih.gov/Disorders/Patient-Caregiver-Education/Fact-Sheets/Low-Back-Pain-Fact-Sheet. Accessed January 15, 2021.

240. Feldman DE. Risk Factors for the Development of Low Back Pain in Adolescence. *Am J Epidemiol.* 2001;154(1):30-36. doi:10.1093/aje/154.1.30

241. Han H Il, Choi HS, Shin WS. Effects of hamstring stretch with pelvic control on pain and work ability in standing workers. *J Back Musculoskelet Rehabil.* 2016;29(4):865-871. doi:10.3233/BMR-160703

242. Witvrouw E, Mahieu N, Danneels L, McNair P. Stretching and injury prevention: An obscure relationship. *Sport Med.* 2004;34(7):443-449. doi:10.2165/00007256-200434070-00003

243. Gartley RM, Lynn Prosser J. Stretching to Prevent Musculoskeletal Injuries An Approach to Workplace Wellness. doi:10.3928/08910162-20110516-02

244. Lee IM, Skerrett PJ. Physical activity and all-cause mortality: What is the dose-response relation? In: *Medicine and Science in Sports and Exercise.* Vol 33. American College of Sports Medicine; 2001. doi:10.1097/00005768-200106001-00016

245. Diet Tool: Calories Burned Calculator for Common Exercises and Activities. https://www.webmd.com/fitness-

exercise/healthtool-exercise-calculator. Accessed
January 15, 2021.

246. How much physical activity do adults need? |
Physical Activity | CDC.
https://www.cdc.gov/physicalactivity/basics/adults
/index.htm. Accessed January 15, 2021.

247. American Heart Association Recommendations for
Physical Activity in Adults and Kids | American
Heart Association.
https://www.heart.org/en/healthy-
living/fitness/fitness-basics/aha-recs-for-physical-
activity-in-adults. Accessed January 15, 2021.

248. MET-hour equivalents of various physical activities -
Harvard Health.
https://www.health.harvard.edu/staying-
healthy/met-hour-equivalents-of-various-physical-
activities. Accessed March 25, 2021.

249. Exercise - NHS. https://www.nhs.uk/live-
well/exercise/. Accessed March 25, 2021.

250. Larson-Meyer DE. A Systematic Review of the Energy
Cost and Metabolic Intensity of Yoga. *Med Sci Sports
Exerc.* 2016;48(8):1558-1569.
doi:10.1249/MSS.0000000000000922

251. Measuring Physical Activity Intensity | Physical
Activity | CDC.
https://www.cdc.gov/physicalactivity/basics/measu
ring/index.html. Accessed March 25, 2021.

252. Burke LE, Ma J, Azar KMJ, et al. Current Science on
Consumer Use of Mobile Health for Cardiovascular
Disease Prevention: A Scientific Statement from the
American Heart Association. *Circulation.*
2015;132(12):1157-1213.
doi:10.1161/CIR.0000000000000232

253. Pollan M. *In Defense of Food: An Eaters's Manifesto.* New

York: Penguin Group; 2008.

254. The most popular diets from the past.
https://www.businessinsider.com/most-popular-
diets-from-the-past-2018-1#2015-whole-30-28.
Accessed February 11, 2021.

255. Jahns L, Davis-Shaw W, Lichtenstein AH, Murphy SP,
Conrad Z, Nielsen F. The history and future of dietary
guidance in America. *Adv Nutr.* 2018;9(2):136-147.
doi:10.1093/advances/nmx025

256. Previous Editions | Dietary Guidelines for Americans.
https://www.dietaryguidelines.gov/about-dietary-
guidelines/previous-editions. Accessed February 11,
2021.

257. Gov D. *Dietary Guidelines for Americans Make Every Bite
Count With the Dietary Guidelines.* https://www.
Accessed February 11, 2021.

258. Hajjar I, Kotchen JM, Kotchen TA. HYPERTENSION:
Trends in Prevalence, Incidence, and Control. *Annu
Rev Public Health.* 2006;27(1):465-490.
doi:10.1146/annurev.publhealth.27.021405.102132

259. Products - Data Briefs - Number 364 - April 2020.
https://www.cdc.gov/nchs/products/databriefs/db
364.htm. Accessed February 11, 2021.

260. for Disease Control C, of Diabetes Translation D. *Long-
Term Trends in Diabetes.*; 2017.
http://www.cdc.gov/diabetes/data. Accessed
February 11, 2021.

261. NCHS Data Visualization Gallery - Mortality Trends in
the United States. https://www.cdc.gov/nchs/data-
visualization/mortality-trends/index.htm. Accessed
February 11, 2021.

262. 4 Total Caloric Intake - Diet, Nutrition, and Cancer -
NCBI Bookshelf.
https://www.ncbi.nlm.nih.gov/books/NBK216632/.

Accessed February 25, 2021.

263. Poti JM, Mendez MA, Ng SW, Popkin BM. Is the degree of food processing and convenience linked with the nutritional quality of foods purchased by US households? *Am J Clin Nutr.* 2015;101(6):1251-1262. doi:10.3945/ajcn.114.100925

264. Can Eating Fruits and Veggies Lower Alzheimer's Risk? https://www.medscape.org/viewarticle/926523_2. Accessed May 5, 2021.

265. News release: Time to curb our appetite for ultra-processed food | Heart and Stroke Foundation. https://www.heartandstroke.ca/what-we-do/media-centre/news-releases/time-to-curb-our-appetite-for-ultra-processed-food. Accessed February 25, 2021.

266. Srour B, Fezeu LK, Kesse-Guyot E, et al. Ultra-processed food intake and risk of cardiovascular disease: Prospective cohort study (NutriNet-Santé). *BMJ.* 2019;365. doi:10.1136/bmj.l1451

267. Rico-Campà A, Martínez-González MA, Alvarez-Alvarez I, et al. Association between consumption of ultra-processed foods and all cause mortality: SUN prospective cohort study. *BMJ.* 2019;365. doi:10.1136/bmj.l1949

268. Ultra-processed food linked to early death - BBC News. https://www.bbc.com/news/health-48446924. Accessed February 25, 2021.

269. Putnam J, Allshouse J, Kantor LS. U.S. Per Capita Food Supply Trends: More Calories, Refined Carbohydrates, and Fats. *FoodReview.* 2002;25(3).

270. O'Hearn M, Liu J, Cudhea F, Micha R, Mozaffarian D. Coronavirus Disease 2019 Hospitalizations Attributable to Cardiometabolic Conditions in the United States: A Comparative Risk Assessment

Analysis. *J Am Heart Assoc.* 2021;10:e019259.
doi:10.1161/JAHA.120.019259

271. Weindruch R, Sohal RS. Caloric Intake and Aging. *N Engl J Med.* 1997;337(14):986-994.
doi:10.1056/nejm199710023371407

272. Gov D. *Dietary Guidelines for Americans Make Every Bite Count With the Dietary Guidelines.* https://www. Accessed February 27, 2021.

273. *How Much Sugar Do You Eat? You May Be Surprised! Added Sugars.* www.dhhs.nh.gov. Accessed February 27, 2021.

274. Fraser GE. Vegetarian diets: What do we know of their effects on common chronic diseases? In: *American Journal of Clinical Nutrition.* Vol 89. American Society for Nutrition; 2009:1607S.
doi:10.3945/ajcn.2009.26736K

275. Still No Free Lunch: Nutrient Levels in U.S. Food Supply Eroded by Pursuit of High Yields | The Organic Center. https://organic-center.org/still-no-free-lunch-nutrient-levels-us-food-supply-eroded-pursuit-high-yields. Accessed January 30, 2021.

276. Davis DR, Epp MD, Riordan HD, Davis DR. Changes in USDA Food Composition Data for 43 Garden Crops, 1950 to 1999. *J Am Coll Nutr.* 2004;23(6):669-682.
doi:10.1080/07315724.2004.10719409

277. Organic foods contain higher levels of certain nutrients, lower levels of pesticides, and may provide health benefits for the consumer - PubMed. https://pubmed.ncbi.nlm.nih.gov/20359265/. Accessed February 27, 2021.

278. Vigar, Myers, Oliver, Arellano, Robinson, Leifert. A Systematic Review of Organic Versus Conventional Food Consumption: Is There a Measurable Benefit on Human Health? *Nutrients.* 2019;12(1):7.

doi:10.3390/nu12010007

279. Zhong VW, Van Horn L, Greenland P, et al. Associations of Processed Meat, Unprocessed Red Meat, Poultry, or Fish Intake with Incident Cardiovascular Disease and All-Cause Mortality. *JAMA Intern Med.* 2020;180(4):503-512. doi:10.1001/jamainternmed.2019.6969

280. Daley CA, Abbott A, Doyle PS, Nader GA, Larson S. A review of fatty acid profiles and antioxidant content in grass-fed and grain-fed beef. *Nutr J.* 2010;9(1):10. doi:10.1186/1475-2891-9-10

281. Fish Faceoff: Wild Salmon vs. Farmed Salmon – Health Essentials from Cleveland Clinic. https://health.clevelandclinic.org/fish-faceoff-wild-salmon-vs-farmed-salmon/. Accessed February 27, 2021.

282. U.S. Food Expenditures at Home and Abroad. https://www.fb.org/market-intel/u.s.-food-expenditures-at-home-and-abroad. Accessed February 27, 2021.

283. How has U.S. spending on healthcare changed over time? - Peterson-KFF Health System Tracker. https://www.healthsystemtracker.org/chart-collection/u-s-spending-healthcare-changed-time/#item-usspendingovertime_3. Accessed May 5, 2021.

284. Handler J. Hypertensive urgency. *J Clin Hypertens (Greenwich).* 2006;8(1):61-64. doi:10.1111/j.1524-6175.2005.05145.x

285. Kumar V, Abbas A, Fausto N, Mtchell R. *Robbins Basic Pathology.* 8th ed. Philadelphia: Saunders Elsevier; 2007.

286. Hypertension Prevalence and Control Among Adults. https://www.cdc.gov/nchs/data/databriefs/db289.p

df. Accessed May 14, 2020.

287. Hypertension. https://www.who.int/news-room/fact-sheets/detail/hypertension. Accessed April 5, 2021.

288. Products - Data Briefs - Number 193 - March 2015. https://www.cdc.gov/nchs/products/databriefs/db193.htm. Accessed May 14, 2020.

289. End Organ Damage In Hypertension. https://www.ncbi.nlm.nih.gov/pmc/articles/PMC3011179/. Accessed May 15, 2020.

290. Willey JZ, Moon YP, Kahn E, et al. Population attributable risks of hypertension and diabetes for cardiovascular disease and stroke in the Northern Manhattan study. *J Am Heart Assoc*. 2014;3(5). doi:10.1161/JAHA.114.001106

291. Aigner A, Grittner U, Rolfs A, Norrving B, Siegerink B, Busch MA. Contribution of Established Stroke Risk Factors to the Burden of Stroke in Young Adults. *Stroke*. 2017;48(7):1744-1751. doi:10.1161/STROKEAHA.117.016599

292. Ruigrok YM, Buskens E, Rinkel GJE. Attributable Risk of Common and Rare Determinants of Subarachnoid Hemorrhage. *Stroke*. 2001;32(5):1173-1175. doi:10.1161/01.STR.32.5.1173

293. Risk factors for myocardial infarction in women and men: insights from the INTERHEART study | European Heart Journal | Oxford Academic. https://academic.oup.com/eurheartj/article/29/7/932/482737. Accessed May 15, 2020.

294. Chronic Kidney Disease in the United States, 2019. https://www.cdc.gov/kidneydisease/publications-resources/2019-national-facts.html?utm_source=miragenews&utm_medium=miragenews&utm_campaign=news. Accessed May 15,

2020.

295. Brandes A, Smit MD, Nguyen BO, Rienstra M, Van Gelder IC. Risk factor management in atrial fibrillation. *Arrhythmia Electrophysiol Rev.* 2018;7(2):118-127. doi:10.15420/aer.2018.18.2

296. Kannel WB. Incidence and epidemiology of heart failure. *Heart Fail Rev.* 2000;5(2):167-173. doi:10.1023/A:1009884820941

297. Vidal-Petiot E, Ford I, Greenlaw N, et al. Cardiovascular event rates and mortality according to achieved systolic and diastolic blood pressure in patients with stable coronary artery disease: an international cohort study. *Lancet.* 2016;388(10056):2142-2152. doi:10.1016/S0140-6736(16)31326-5

298. Pellerito J, Polak J. *Introduction to Vascular Ultrasonography.* 6th ed. Philadelphia: Elsevier Saunders; 2012.

299. Know Your Risk for High Blood Pressure | cdc.gov. https://www.cdc.gov/bloodpressure/risk_factors.htm. Accessed May 15, 2020.

300. Beevers G, Lip GYH, O'brien E. The pathophysiology of hypertension. *BMJ.* 2001;322(7291):912. doi:10.1136/bmj.322.7291.912

301. Alexander RW. Hypertension and the Pathogenesis of Atherosclerosis. *Hypertension.* 1995;25(2):155-161. doi:10.1161/01.HYP.25.2.155

302. Rafieian-Kopaei M, Setorki M, Doudi M, Baradaran A, Nasri H. Atherosclerosis: Process, indicators, risk factors and new hopes. *Int J Prev Med.* 2014;5(8):927-946.

303. Bidani AK, Griffin KA. Pathophysiology of hypertensive renal damage: Implications for therapy. *Hypertension.* 2004;44(5):595-601.

doi:10.1161/01.HYP.0000145180.38707.84

304. Products - Data Briefs - Number 278 - April 2017. https://www.cdc.gov/nchs/products/databriefs/db 278.htm. Accessed May 15, 2020.

305. Heart-Health Screenings | American Heart Association. https://www.heart.org/en/health-topics/consumer-healthcare/what-is-cardiovascular-disease/heart-health-screenings. Accessed May 17, 2020.

306. Schwartz CL, McManus RJ. What is the evidence base for diagnosing hypertension and for subsequent blood pressure treatment targets in the prevention of cardiovascular disease? *BMC Med.* 2015;13(1):256. doi:10.1186/s12916-015-0502-5

307. Monitoring Your Blood Pressure at Home | American Heart Association. https://www.heart.org/en/health-topics/high-blood-pressure/understanding-blood-pressure-readings/monitoring-your-blood-pressure-at-home. Accessed May 17, 2020.

308. How Accurate Are Blood Pressure Machine Readings? – CBS Pittsburgh. https://pittsburgh.cbslocal.com/2013/11/22/how-accurate-are-blood-pressure-machine-readings/. Accessed May 17, 2020.

309. Whitcomb BL, Prochazka A, Loverde M, Byyny RL. Failure of the Community-Based Vita-Stat Automated Blood Pressure Device to Accurately Measure Blood Pressure. *Arch Fam Med.* 1995;4(5):419-424. doi:10.1001/archfami.4.5.419

310. Lewis JE, Boyle E, Magharious L, Myers MG. Evaluation of a community-based automated blood pressure measuring device. *C Can Med Assoc J.* 2002;166(9):1145.

311. Do community based self-reading sphygmomanometers improve detection of hypertension? A feasibility study. - PubMed - NCBI. https://www.ncbi.nlm.nih.gov/pubmed/12848401. Accessed May 17, 2020.

312. Berra E, Azizi M, Capron A, et al. Evaluation of Adherence Should Become an Integral Part of Assessment of Patients with Apparently Treatment-Resistant Hypertension. *Hypertension*. 2016;68(2):297-306. doi:10.1161/HYPERTENSIONAHA.116.07464

313. 8 reasons patients don't take their medications | American Medical Association. https://www.ama-assn.org/delivering-care/patient-support-advocacy/8-reasons-patients-dont-take-their-medications. Accessed May 15, 2020.

314. Bureau UC. Age and Sex Composition in the United States: 2019. https://www.census.gov/data/tables/2019/demo/age-and-sex/2019-age-sex-composition.html. Accessed November 4, 2021.

315. Lifestyle changes reduce the need for blood pressure medications | American Heart Association. https://newsroom.heart.org/news/lifestyle-changes-reduce-the-need-for-blood-pressure-medications?preview=3b29. Accessed May 15, 2020.

316. Early History of Cancer | American Cancer Society. https://www.cancer.org/cancer/cancer-basics/history-of-cancer/what-is-cancer.html. Accessed April 30, 2020.

317. Cancer is the leading cause of death in dogs and cats. http://www.vetcontact.com/en/art.php?a=773. Accessed April 30, 2020.

318. Fibrosarcoma in Birds - Symptoms, Causes, Diagnosis, Treatment, Recovery, Management, Cost.

https://wagwalking.com/bird/condition/fibrosarcoma. Accessed April 5, 2021.

319. Cancer in Wild Animals | CancerQuest. https://www.cancerquest.org/cancer-biology/cancer-wild-animals. Accessed April 30, 2020.

320. Cell Division, Cancer | Learn Science at Scitable. https://www.nature.com/scitable/topicpage/cell-division-and-cancer-14046590/. Accessed April 30, 2020.

321. End-of-Life Care - National Cancer Institute. https://www.cancer.gov/about-cancer/advanced-cancer/care-choices/care-fact-sheet. Accessed April 30, 2020.

322. Cancer Staging - National Cancer Institute. https://www.cancer.gov/about-cancer/diagnosis-staging/staging. Accessed April 30, 2020.

323. Survival Rates for Breast Cancer. https://www.cancer.org/cancer/breast-cancer/understanding-a-breast-cancer-diagnosis/breast-cancer-survival-rates.html. Accessed April 30, 2020.

324. Cancer Screening Guidelines | Detecting Cancer Early. https://www.cancer.org/healthy/find-cancer-early/cancer-screening-guidelines/american-cancer-society-guidelines-for-the-early-detection-of-cancer.html. Accessed May 1, 2020.

325. Topic Search Results | United States Preventive Services Taskforce. https://uspreventiveservicestaskforce.org/uspstf/topic_search_results?topic_status=P. Accessed May 1, 2020.

326. Cancer Screening Tests | CDC. https://www.cdc.gov/cancer/dcpc/prevention/screening.htm. Accessed May 1, 2020.

327. Cancer Screening Overview (PDQ®)–Patient Version - National Cancer Institute. https://www.cancer.gov/about-cancer/screening/patient-screening-overview-pdq. Accessed May 1, 2020.

328. Breast Cancer Screening for Women at Average Risk: 2015 Guideline Update from the American Cancer Society. https://www.ncbi.nlm.nih.gov/pmc/articles/PMC4831582/. Accessed May 1, 2020.

329. (No Title). https://www.cancer.org/content/dam/cancer-org/research/cancer-facts-and-statistics/annual-cancer-facts-and-figures/2020/cancer-facts-and-figures-2020.pdf. Accessed March 2, 2020.

330. Cervical Cancer — Cancer Stat Facts. https://seer.cancer.gov/statfacts/html/cervix.html. Accessed May 2, 2020.

331. Pinkbook | HPV | Epidemiology of Vaccine Preventable Diseases | CDC. https://www.cdc.gov/vaccines/pubs/pinkbook/hpv.html. Accessed May 2, 2020.

332. The HPV Vaccine: Access and Use in the U.S. | The Henry J. Kaiser Family Foundation. https://www.kff.org/womens-health-policy/fact-sheet/the-hpv-vaccine-access-and-use-in-the-u-s/. Accessed July 25, 2021.

333. Colorectal Cancer: Screening | Recommendation | United States Preventive Services Taskforce. https://www.uspreventiveservicestaskforce.org/uspstf/recommendation/colorectal-cancer-screening#fig. Accessed May 4, 2020.

334. Family Health History of Colorectal (Colon) Cancer | CDC.

https://www.cdc.gov/genomics/disease/colorectal_cancer/family_history_coloretal.htm. Accessed May 4, 2020.

335. He J, Efron JE. Screening for Colorectal Cancer. *Adv Surg.* 2011;45(1):31-44. doi:10.1016/j.yasu.2011.03.006

336. Richards TB, Doria-Rose VP, Soman A, et al. Lung Cancer Screening Inconsistent With U.S. Preventive Services Task Force Recommendations. *Am J Prev Med.* 2019;56(1):66-73. doi:10.1016/j.amepre.2018.07.030

337. Prostate-Specific Antigen (PSA) Test - National Cancer Institute. https://www.cancer.gov/types/prostate/psa-fact-sheet#what-is-a-normal-psa-test-result. Accessed May 4, 2020.

338. Prostate Cancer: Screening | Recommendation | United States Preventive Services Taskforce. https://www.uspreventiveservicestaskforce.org/uspstf/recommendation/prostate-cancer-screening. Accessed May 4, 2020.

339. Neurologic Complications of Prostate Cancer - American Family Physician. https://www.aafp.org/afp/2002/0501/p1834.html. Accessed May 4, 2020.

340. Prostate Cancer Screening and Early Detection. https://www.pcf.org/about-prostate-cancer/diagnosis-staging-prostate-cancer/screening-early-detection/. Accessed May 4, 2020.

341. Wallis CJD, Haider MA, Nam RK. Role of mpMRI of the prostate in screening for prostate cancer. *Transl Androl Urol.* 2017;6(3):464-471. doi:10.21037/tau.2017.04.31

342. Cascella M, Rajnik M, Cuomo A, Dulebohn SC, Di Napoli R. *Features, Evaluation and Treatment Coronavirus (COVID-19).* StatPearls Publishing; 2020.

http://www.ncbi.nlm.nih.gov/pubmed/32150360.
Accessed April 15, 2020.

343. Timeline: How the Wuhan lab-leak theory suddenly
became credible - The Washington Post.
https://www.washingtonpost.com/politics/2021/05
/25/timeline-how-wuhan-lab-leak-theory-suddenly-
became-credible/. Accessed June 16, 2021.

344. WHO Coronavirus (COVID-19) Dashboard | WHO
Coronavirus (COVID-19) Dashboard With Vaccination
Data.
https://covid19.who.int/?adgroupsurvey=%7Badgro
upsurvey%7D&gclid=EAIaIQobChMIlqGS7qzP7wIV
CxmtBh0K9Q4iEAAYASABEgKnufD_BwE. Accessed
June 16, 2021.

345. CDC COVID Data Tracker.
https://covid.cdc.gov/covid-data-
tracker/#datatracker-home. Accessed June 16, 2021.

346. How many jobs were lost in 2020 due to COVID-19? |
World Economic Forum.
https://www.weforum.org/agenda/2021/02/covid-
employment-global-job-loss/. Accessed March 26,
2021.

347. 8 Million Americans Fell Below the Poverty Line Over
the Past 5 Months.
https://www.businessinsider.com/how-many-
americans-fell-into-poverty-during-pandemic-2020-12.
Accessed March 26, 2021.

348. Updated estimates of the impact of COVID-19 on
global poverty: Looking back at 2020 and the outlook
for 2021.
https://blogs.worldbank.org/opendata/updated-
estimates-impact-covid-19-global-poverty-looking-
back-2020-and-outlook-2021. Accessed March 26, 2021.

349. With record-setting speed, vaccinemakers take their

first shots at the new coronavirus | Science | AAAS.
https://www.sciencemag.org/news/2020/03/record-setting-speed-vaccine-makers-take-their-first-shots-new-coronavirus. Accessed April 15, 2020.

350. NIH Clinical Trial of Investigational Vaccine for COVID-19 Begins | NIH: National Institute of Allergy and Infectious Diseases. https://www.niaid.nih.gov/news-events/nih-clinical-trial-investigational-vaccine-covid-19-begins. Accessed April 15, 2020.

351. Here Are All the Companies Working on COVID-19 Vaccines, Treatments, and Testing. https://www.fool.com/investing/2020/04/07/here-are-all-the-companies-working-on-covid-19-vac.aspx. Accessed April 15, 2020.

352. Learn More About COVID-19 Vaccines From the FDA | FDA. https://www.fda.gov/consumers/consumer-updates/learn-more-about-covid-19-vaccines-fda. Accessed April 5, 2021.

353. CDC COVID Data Tracker. https://covid.cdc.gov/covid-data-tracker/#vaccinations. Accessed June 16, 2021.

354. Hussain A, Ali S, Ahmed M, Hussain S. The Anti-vaccination Movement: A Regression in Modern Medicine. *Cureus*. 2018;10(7). doi:10.7759/cureus.2919

355. Vaccine Myths Debunked | PublicHealth.org. https://www.publichealth.org/public-awareness/understanding-vaccines/vaccine-myths-debunked/. Accessed April 15, 2020.

356. (No Title). https://www.ncbi.nlm.nih.gov/pmc/articles/PMC2831678/pdf/182e199.pdf. Accessed April 15, 2020.

357. BMJ: Wakefield Paper Alleging Link between MMR Vaccine and Autism Fraudulent | History of Vaccines.

https://www.historyofvaccines.org/content/blog/b
mj-wakefield-paper-alleging-link-between-mmr-
vaccine-and-autism-fraudulent. Accessed April 15,
2020.

358. Vaccines Do Not Cause Autism | Concerns | Vaccine
Safety | CDC.
https://www.cdc.gov/vaccinesafety/concerns/autis
m.html. Accessed April 15, 2020.

359. Support for Vaccines Continues Downward Trend in
US, Poll Shows.
https://www.medscape.com/viewarticle/923920?nli
d=133600_436&src=WNL_mdplsfeat_200121_mscpedi
t_publ&uac=170929SJ&spon=42&impID=2252132&faf
=1. Accessed April 15, 2020.

360. Kuehn B. Unvaccinated Children. *JAMA*.
2018;320(20):2069. doi:10.1001/jama.2018.17829

361. Achievements in Public Health, 1900-1999 Impact of
Vaccines Universally Recommended for Children --
United States, 1990-1998.
https://www.cdc.gov/mmwr/preview/mmwrhtml/
00056803.htm. Accessed April 15, 2020.

362. Stratton K, Ford A, Rusch E, Clayton EW. *Adverse
Effects of Vaccines: Evidence and Causality*. National
Academies Press; 2012. doi:10.17226/13164

363. Families I of M (US) C on P and E-LC for C and T,
Field MJ, Behrman RE. PATTERNS OF CHILDHOOD
DEATH IN AMERICA. 2003.
https://www.ncbi.nlm.nih.gov/books/NBK220806/.
Accessed June 16, 2021.

364. Measles | History of Measles | CDC.
https://www.cdc.gov/measles/about/history.html.
Accessed April 15, 2020.

365. The world before vaccines is a world we can't afford to
forget.

https://www.nationalgeographic.com/culture/article
/cannot-forget-world-before-vaccines. Accessed June
16, 2021.

366. WHO EMRO | Disease burden | Haemophilus
influenzae type B | Health topics.
http://www.emro.who.int/health-
topics/haemophilus-influenzae-type-b/disease-
burden.html. Accessed October 20, 2021.

367. More than 140,000 die from measles as cases surge
worldwide. https://www.who.int/news/item/05-12-
2019-more-than-140-000-die-from-measles-as-cases-
surge-worldwide. Accessed October 20, 2021.

368. Measles Outbreak — California, December 2014–
February 2015.
https://www.cdc.gov/mmwr/preview/mmwrhtml/
mm6406a5.htm. Accessed April 15, 2020.

369. Vaccine refusal helped fuel Disneyland measles
outbreak, study says - Los Angeles Times.
https://www.latimes.com/science/sciencenow/la-
sci-sn-disneyland-measles-under-vaccination-
20150316-story.html. Accessed April 15, 2020.

370. Past Seasons Estimated Influenza Disease Burden |
CDC. https://www.cdc.gov/flu/about/burden/past-
seasons.html. Accessed April 15, 2020.

371. Frequently Asked Questions about Estimated Flu
Burden | CDC.
https://www.cdc.gov/flu/about/burden/faq.htm.
Accessed April 15, 2020.

372. Summary of the 2017-2018 Influenza Season | CDC.
https://www.cdc.gov/flu/about/season/flu-season-
2017-2018.htm. Accessed April 15, 2020.

373. Past Seasons Estimated Influenza Disease Burden
Averted by Vaccination | CDC.
https://www.cdc.gov/flu/vaccines-work/past-

burden-averted-est.html. Accessed April 15, 2020.

374. Varicella.
https://www.cdc.gov/vaccines/pubs/pinkbook/do
wnloads/varicella.pdf. Accessed May 19, 2020.

375. Chickenpox Vaccination | What You Should Know |
CDC.
https://www.cdc.gov/vaccines/vpd/varicella/publi
c/index.html. Accessed May 19, 2020.

376. Vaccine Types | Vaccines.
https://www.vaccines.gov/basics/types. Accessed
May 20, 2020.

377. Vaccine Ingredients | Vaccines.
https://www.vaccines.gov/basics/vaccine_ingredien
ts. Accessed May 20, 2020.

378. Vaccine Safety | Vaccines.
https://www.vaccines.gov/basics/safety. Accessed
May 20, 2020.

379. Taylor LE, Swerdfeger AL, Eslick GD. Vaccines are not
associated with autism: An evidence-based meta-
analysis of case-control and cohort studies. *Vaccine*.
2014;32(29):3623-3629.
doi:10.1016/j.vaccine.2014.04.085

380. Destefano F, Price CS, Weintraub ES. Increasing
Exposure to Antibody-Stimulating Proteins and
Polysaccharides in Vaccines Is Not Associated with
Risk of Autism AD Autistic disorder ADI-R Autism
Diagnostic Interview-Revised ADOS Autism
Diagnostic Observation Schedule ASD Autism
spectrum disorder MCO Managed care organization
SCQ Social Communication Questionnaire. 2013.
doi:10.1016/j.jpeds.2013.02.001

381. Gerber JS, Offit PA. Vaccines and autism: A tale of
shifting hypotheses. *Clin Infect Dis*. 2009;48(4):456-461.
doi:10.1086/596476

382. Vaccine Adverse Events: Separating Myth from Reality - American Family Physician. https://www.aafp.org/afp/2017/0615/p786.html#af p20170615p786-b70. Accessed May 20, 2020.

383. Pellegrino P, Carnovale C, Perrone V, et al. Acute Disseminated Encephalomyelitis Onset: Evaluation Based on Vaccine Adverse Events Reporting Systems. *PLoS One*. 2013;8(10). doi:10.1371/journal.pone.0077766

384. HRSA Data and Statistics. https://www.hrsa.gov/sites/default/files/hrsa/vacc ine-compensation/monthly-website-stats-2-01-18.pdf. Published 2018. Accessed May 20, 2020.

385. INFLAMMATORY/POST-INFECTIOUS ENCEPHALOMYELITIS | Journal of Neurology, Neurosurgery & Psychiatry. https://jnnp.bmj.com/content/75/suppl_1/i22. Accessed May 20, 2020.

386. Chen Y, Ma F, Xu Y, Chu X, Zhang J. Vaccines and the risk of acute disseminated encephalomyelitis. *Vaccine*. 2018;36(26):3733-3739. doi:10.1016/j.vaccine.2018.05.063

387. Al Qudah Z, Abukwaik W, Patel H, Souayah N. Encephalitis after Vaccination in United States. A Report from the CDC/FDA Vaccine Adverse Event Reporting System. [1990–2010] (P03.151). *Neurology*. 2012;78(1 Supplement).

388. Guillain-Barré Syndrome Concerns | Vaccine Safety | CDC. https://www.cdc.gov/vaccinesafety/concerns/guilla in-barre-syndrome.html. Accessed May 20, 2020.

389. Investigation of the Temporal Association of Guillain-Barre Syndrome With Influenza Vaccine and Influenzalike Illness Using the United Kingdom

General Practice Research Database - PubMed.
https://pubmed.ncbi.nlm.nih.gov/19033158/.
Accessed May 20, 2020.

390. Kwong JC, Vasa PP, Campitelli MA, et al. Risk of
Guillain-Barré syndrome after seasonal influenza
vaccination and influenza health-care encounters: A
self-controlled study. *Lancet Infect Dis.* 2013;13(9):769-
776. doi:10.1016/S1473-3099(13)70104-X

391. Cecinati V, Principi N, Brescia L, Giordano P, Esposito
S. Vaccine administration and the development of
immune thrombocytopenic purpura in children. *Hum
Vaccines Immunother.* 2013;9(5):1158-1162.
doi:10.4161/hv.23601

392. Vaccines are safe | National Academies.
https://sites.nationalacademies.org/BasedOnScience
/vaccines-are-safe/index.htm. Accessed April 15,
2020.

393. Lightning Strike Victim Data | Lightning | CDC.
https://www.cdc.gov/disasters/lightning/victimdat
a.html. Accessed April 5, 2021.

394. Ahmad FB, Anderson RN. The Leading Causes of
Death in the US for 2020. *JAMA - J Am Med Assoc.*
2021;325(18):1829-1830. doi:10.1001/jama.2021.5469

395. HSF.
https://spaceflight.nasa.gov/shuttle/upgrades/upgr
ades5.html. Accessed January 31, 2021.

396. Bianconi E, Piovesan A, Facchin F, et al. An estimation
of the number of cells in the human body. *Ann Hum
Biol.* 2013;40(6):463-471.
doi:10.3109/03014460.2013.807878

397. How many organs are in the human body? | Live
Science. https://www.livescience.com/how-many-

organs-in-human-body.html. Accessed January 31, 2021.

398. Sender R, Fuchs S, Milo R. Revised Estimates for the Number of Human and Bacteria Cells in the Body. *PLoS Biol*. 2016;14(8). doi:10.1371/journal.pbio.1002533

About the Author

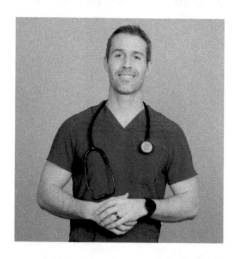

Dr. Ramirez is a Vascular Neurologist specializing in the prevention and treatment of neurologic emergencies such as strokes and brain hemorrhages. Growing up, he never envisioned of becoming a doctor, though his admiration of the human body while studying anatomy in college lead him down the path of becoming the first physician in his family. Trained at renowned academic institutions in Los Angeles, he now works in Southern California at one of the most reputable hospital systems in the nation. Importantly to him, his experiences ignited a passion for stroke prevention, driving him to integrate disease prevention and community education into his practice.

Note from the Author

Word-of-mouth is crucial for any author to succeed. If you enjoyed *Simplify Your Health*, please leave a review online — anywhere you are able. Even if it's just a sentence or two. It would make all the difference and would be very much appreciated.

Thanks!
Lucas Ramirez, MD

We hope you enjoyed reading this title from:

BLACK ROSE
writing™

www.blackrosewriting.com

Subscribe to our mailing list – *The Rosevine* – and receive **FREE** books, daily deals, and stay current with news about upcoming releases and our hottest authors.
Scan the QR code below to sign up.

Already a subscriber? Please accept a sincere thank you for being a fan of Black Rose Writing authors.

View other Black Rose Writing titles at
www.blackrosewriting.com/books and use promo code
PRINT to receive a **20% discount** when purchasing.

CPSIA information can be obtained
at www.ICGtesting.com
Printed in the USA
BVHW030606190722
642003BV00004B/13